Narratives of Narcolepsy in Everyday Life

LEXINGTON STUDIES IN HEALTH COMMUNICATION

Series Editors: Leandra H. Hernández and Kari Nixon

National and international governments have recognized the importance of widespread, timely, and effective health communication, as research shows that accurate, patient-centered, and culturally competent health communication can improve patient and community health care outcomes. This interdisciplinary series examines the role of health communication in society and is receptive to manuscripts and edited volumes that use a variety of theoretical, methodological, interdisciplinary, and intersectional approaches. We invite contributions on a variety of health communication topics including but not limited to health communication in a digital age; race, gender, ethnicity, class, physical abilities, and health communication; critical approaches to health communication; feminisms and health communication; LGBTQIA health; interpersonal health communication perspectives; rhetorical approaches to health communication; organizational approaches to health communication; health campaigns, media effects, and health communication; multicultural approaches to health communication; and international health communication. This series is open to contributions from scholars representing communication, women's and gender studies, public health, health education, discursive analyses of medical rhetoric, and other disciplines whose work interrogates and explores these topics. Successful proposals will be accessible to an interdisciplinary audience, advance our understanding of contemporary approaches to health communication, and enrich our conversations about the importance of health communication in today's health landscape.

Recent Titles in This Series

Narratives of Narcolepsy in Everyday Life: Exploring Intricacies of Identity, Sleepiness, and Place, by Nicole Eugene

A Culturally Centered and Intersectional Approach to Reproductive Justice, edited by Tomeka M. Robinson, Sabrina Singh, and Christina Mary Joseph

PCOS Discourses, Symbolic Impacts, and Feminist Rhetorical Disruptions of Institutional Hegemonies, by Marissa C. McKinley

Narratives of Narcolepsy in Everyday Life

Exploring Intricacies of Identity, Sleepiness, and Place

Nicole Eugene

LEXINGTON BOOKS
Lanham • Boulder • New York • London

Published by Lexington Books
An imprint of The Rowman & Littlefield Publishing Group, Inc.
4501 Forbes Boulevard, Suite 200, Lanham, Maryland 20706
www.rowman.com

86-90 Paul Street, London EC2A 4NE, United Kingdom

British Library Cataloguing in Publication Information Available

Library of Congress Cataloging-in-Publication Data Available

ISBN 978-1-66691-318-7 (cloth : alk. paper) | ISBN 978-1-66691-319-4 (ebook)

Contents

Preface

In one sense, this project began over twenty years ago when I was diagnosed with narcolepsy at the age of sixteen. The letter the sleep specialist wrote to my primary care doctor memorializes this day beginning with these words: "Thank you for asking me to see this interesting sixteen-year-old black female with daytime somnolence." The letter, dated October 15, 1996, goes on to explain that the sleep test and genetic test confirmed the diagnosis of narcolepsy before moving on to describe the prescribed treatment that would be adjusted monthly until we found the appropriate dosage of stimulants. During those first months after my diagnosis, I went to our encyclopedia and looked up narcolepsy and mused at the way the author was both undoubtedly negative about what life with narcolepsy meant while also praising the intelligence of people with narcolepsy. In the months and years that followed, the author's offer of pity mixed with praise would revisit me time and again. Like many newly diagnosed people, I was thirsty for information about the condition and was rarely satisfied with what I located—until I asked my mom to buy the book by Marguerite Utley (1995), *Narcolepsy: A Funny Disorder That's No Laughing Matter.* This self-published book combined nonacademic research with personal narrative to provide readers with pragmatic information and moments of companionship. As I flip through the thin paperback now, I see descriptions of symptoms that lack the cultivation and meticulous citationality that book publishers and editors might have required, but I also see the highlighted areas that I carried with me during those twenty plus years—literally, and in the ways the book shaped my view of narcolepsy. Her book greatly enriched my life, and I suspect that it positively affected the lives of many others in the pre–smart phone, pre–2.0 internet, and pre–social media world.

For a long time, Utley's book was the only one written by and for people with narcolepsy. However, when Julie Flygare (2013) published her memoir, *Wide Awake and Dreaming*, which quickly became the most popular book on narcolepsy, the world had transformed. As I write today, there are numerous blogs, video blogs, books, social media platforms, and online forums for people with narcolepsy to learn about this strange and often debilitating condition. With all these highly visible narratives of narcolepsy, how can I present research on life with narcolepsy in a novel light? Moreover, are there better ways to communicate about narcolepsy that can help others empathize, understand, and assist—is there a way to communicate about this hidden disability that does not also hide the personal struggles? The present book goes beyond the search for voices and information into a quest to better understand how narratives about everyday life with narcolepsy can create an account of narcolepsy that pays attention to contextual factors shaping the meaning of narcolepsy and its symptoms. By blending methods of inquiry and by experimenting with narrative writing, I approach both the absences narcolepsy creates and the presence it has in everyday life in a way that respects and legitimizes both dimensions of the condition.

This book occupies a unique intersection of perspectives and methods because the subject of narcolepsy, and the spaciotemporal rebels it creates, live in direct opposition to the many cultural dictums that shape the core of everyday life in the United States and many other parts of the world. I also bring a wide range of theories and methodological influences to this project because of my previous work in sociology, folklore, cultural studies, and communication studies. This preface will detail some of the preliminary research and the ideas seeded earlier and are blooming buds in these pages.

Health communication and social support research in the area of disabilities and chronic illnesses tended to cluster around the concepts like disclosure, stigma, and label management. Therefore, I did an exploratory project in which I conducted email interviews with forty-nine people with narcolepsy and asked them questions connected to concepts like stigma, disclosure, and label management. This research revealed that while these are useful concepts, they tended to limit my inquiries to textual and oral representations of health information and did not provide insights into the complexities that characterize efforts to communicate about narcolepsy.

This preliminary project was fruitful in other ways. For example, my initial questions—about what narcolepsy is and how narcolepsy affects interviewees' lives—were intended to build rapport before asking the more difficult questions about disclosure, stigma, and label management. However, for some people these questions were approached as rare opportunities to textually perform their narcolepsy. In other words, in addition to receiving conventional answers, I also received poetry, reenactments of their day, metaphors, and biographical sketches. These were people who wanted to be seen in all their complexity and messiness. My thirteenth interviewee, Mary, provided a memorable answer to the question, "Please tell me a little about what your life is like as a person living with narcolepsy." Mary gave me the short version first, "Short version: It's painful and you feel guilty for not being able to do everything that everyone else does. Your body hurts and you forget a lot. You can't trust your body or your mind." Then she went on for nearly two pages describing a longer answer to the question, beginning with:

> Very long description of a day in my life: The alarm goes off at 5:30 a.m. I wake up and get ready for work and make my lunch 3–5 times each morning before I realize I am still in bed.
>
> 6:00 a.m. But I can't get out of bed yet, I am in too much pain and freezing.
>
> 6:05 a.m. I am able to sit up and walk to the bathroom, I keep the doors open because my hands don't work quite yet.
>
> It's 6:15 a.m.? Did I just fall asleep peeing? I don't remember falling asleep. Better hurry, I am going to be late.
>
> 6:20 a.m. clothes on, hair brushed, now where are my keys? Never mind I'll use the spare set.
>
> 6:22 a.m. Wait, what am I wearing? I can't wear this to work.
>
> 6:25 a.m. change clothes, I have to go NOW.
>
> 6:27 a.m. check on the baby . . . accidently wake up the baby. Oops, sorry honey.
>
> 6:30 a.m. Oh! I need lunch! *open the fridge* There's my car keys!!
>
> 6:32 a.m. Start my car, exit the neighborhood . . .
>
> 6:48 a.m. How did I get to work? I don't remember driving.

This excerpt ends with a reference to automatic behavior, a symptom of narcolepsy that will be briefly discussed in the first two chapters. Mary's vivid account goes far beyond a struggle with getting up in the morning. Her description of making lunch refers to the way dreams and thinking about the morning can trick people with narcolepsy into mistaking sleep for wakefulness. She went on to describe the various ways narcolepsy can affect aspects of executive functioning like memory and attention. As a whole, her response highlighted how the intricacies of everyday life are more than a context, rather they are integral to what each symptom means and what narcolepsy means. Accurate, objective, and medical descriptions of the symptoms or the physiopathology pale in comparison to this striking account. Mary's tiny glimpse into how her day began provides just enough framework for readers to decipher the many ways in which narcolepsy is potentially disabling.

Eve was my first interviewee out of the sample; she was a married woman who had narcolepsy with cataplexy. Since I was at my computer when she sent her initial response, I was able to read her answers immediately and ask follow-up questions. Our email exchange was similar to a conversation because it was occurring in real time and the depth of our exchange reflects this. Even though laughter is a cataplexy trigger for Eve, she works as a part time professional comedian. Curious about why she would put herself in a situation where cataplexy was likely, I asked, "Can you tell me about your relationship to humor? It seems to be a trigger and a way to make hard discussions fun. Also, how did you come to embrace humor the way you have?" To which she replied:

> Allow for a bit of a free flow here, as it's a complicated and paradoxical relationship. My relationship to humor is like an emergency room doctor or [a] mortician's relationship to humor. It's gallows humor. Humor is therapy to help the soul cope with pain. The clown is the saddest of all behind his makeup, and Robin Williams killed himself. To laugh can cut my puppet strings and make me fall, and I am the puppet master causing audiences to laugh. Laughter is the best medicine, but in my case it can be bad medicine. They laugh with me, they laugh at me, I control it I provide it. I am a practitioner of that which causes me pain.

Being able to quickly follow up with her shows how internet interviews can approximate some of the back and forth possible in face-to-face interviews. These exchanges foreshadowed my embrace of a performative or narrative approach used in sharing my exchanges with participants in parts of this book.

By deciding not to share my identity as a person with narcolepsy I hoped to model interpretivist and post-positivist research on stigma and label management in health communication research. After analyzing these and other interviews focusing on issue of disclosure, as I had planned, I realized that I also was performing. By hiding my narcolepsy, I was acting as if I was an objective non-narcoleptic communication researcher. Moreover, it felt dishonest to pretend that I was not an empathetic fellow narcoleptic who was on a parallel sleepy voyage. Despite this ethical tension, the research provided many insights into the complex world of narcolepsy. The experience seeded in me a distaste for approaching people with narcolepsy under what felt like false pretenses. Instead of hiding my identity as someone with narcolepsy, I decided to build on my experiences of doing peer interviews where we exchanged stories. My need to address myself as a racialized subject was similarly about being honest with my readers and myself while also creating a fuller sense of how chronic illness and disability are experienced.

My work with the Surviving Katrina and Rita in Houston Projects with Carl Lindahl at the University of Houston introduced me to the world of narrative from the perspective of folklore (Eugene, 2006; Lindahl, 2012; Lindahl et al., 2009). Folklorists are interested in the stories of ordinary people but not solely as potential data to apply theories. Rather they listen and examine stories because quality stories provide insights into the human dramas that bind all people together. Lindahl also taught me how to listen to my interviewees, to get lost in their worlds, and to go where *they* would like to go. He also introduced me to the peer interview model that also operated as a type of intervention in which people who are experiencing a unique hardship are granted the company of a fellow voyager on their own hardship journey (Lindahl, 2006). There is a clear possibility that one of these people can pull us both under a current of despair and desolation. However, my experience with the process of peer interviewing showed me that instead, we helped each other and affirmed each other's resilience and sense of belonging.

As an unmoored person recently relocated in Houston, I had the opportunity to connect with fellow displaced persons via Dr. Lindahl's interview and archive project. This proved to be an invitation to build community and belonging. The vicissitudes of life with narcolepsy often strain many familial and communal relationships and so this book recounts a parallel invitation for participants and researcher alike. Around this time, as a guest editor for the *Anthropology of Consciousness,* Matt Wolf-Meyer invited me to write autoethnographically about my life with narcolepsy to contribute to its exploration of sleep (Eugene, 2013; M. Wolf-Meyer, 2013). I hastily threw myself into the writing and editing like nothing I had ever done before. Enamored with the writing process, I would get lost in the creative destruction of rewriting and revisions. The editors and reviewers did not request any revisions or edits, which somewhat shocked me. Ever since then autoethnography, or writing as a way to make sense of one's life with the aid of theory, has been a siren that called me to tumultuously rocky shores. Because as much as I savored laboring over words, they also can vex like nothing else. They may often slip through my grasp or worse, as one interviewee exclaimed, they can suddenly fall "out of my head." Similarly, I'm at times drawn towards the emotive power of poetry and performative writing while unceremoniously also running away from it because the shared concrete language of health insurance, doctors, and medication wields a different type of power that operates in my life and the lives of people with chronic illnesses. This book entwines the heart of peer research with the soul of creative research in an attempt to articulate the substances that labor to animate the people who have been touched by narcolepsy.

As a book born of multilayered influences and interdisciplinary roots, it seeks to contribute to health communication in a few ways. Rather than belabor these hopes here, I will instead acknowledge how pleasing it has been to see the decidedly quantitative area of inquiry embrace and partner with critical, rhetorical, and qualitative scholars in recent years, proving its profound capacity for flexibility and adaptation. It is this spirit of flexibility and adaptation that allowed me, a marginalized member of a group, to devise a method for exploring oneself and a community of individuals as they wrestle with the bizarre reality of life with narcolepsy. Life with a potentially stigmatizing and unpredictable condition sets the stage for taking various perspectives on the everyday. I often use the framework of an adventure to marvel at all that has unfolded in a life that some authors expected so little of. Adventures pose challenges and complications that are often met with a measure of uncertainty. Similarly, my attraction to research is rooted in the awe inherent in the experience of uncovering what was not previously known. All of these sensibilities are a part of what brought this book into existence and are woven between the pages and the words.

Acknowledgments

One morning I noticed the sound of a bird persistently chirping outside my patio window. This sound seemed much closer than usual, so I went outside expecting to see a bird attempting to build a nest or something like that. I found something that initially confused me and somewhat surprised me. There were two birds. One was a mahogany adult bird that perched on the patio chair before noisily flying away and back. The other was a small, young fluffy bird, much quieter, on the cement under yard supplies. The smaller bird might have been hiding from me or from something else. After searching online, I learned that the small bird was a fledgling, who was likely learning how to fly or walk and that the parent bird was staying close to provide support and protection. I also learned that if there were no injuries or pet dangers in the area these animals did not need human intervention. The young bird simply needed time to master the skills of flying and walking. When I learned that the noise of the parent bird might remain for a few days I realized that I might get used to it; but after another hour or two silence returned to the patio. They both left, which both saddened and uplifted me.

Many years ago, my brief time as a bookseller and my years as an avid book reader planted in me a determination to get a PhD, become a professor, and to publish a book. This last endeavor turned out to be more difficult than I had initially imagined it to be. I have also changed immeasurably through those years and can thank a large, disperse community of scholars and nonscholars for supporting me and/or my work. Each of the people I have acknowledged here have, in their own way, circled me and supported me like the parent bird did as I developed my confidence and skills as an educator, a researcher, and a writer. I have decided to organize this in chronological order to resemble a story.

Firstly, I would like to express my deep and undying appreciation for my parents and my siblings as people who have supported me in countless ways. My dad's endless curiosity about the world and interest in learning is something I am proud to share with him. I also genuinely appreciate the love, care, and support my mother provided through my younger years, through the Spelman years, and beyond. Despite the countless tiffs I've had with her, Hope Thompson's adolescent love of speech and debate introduced me to a world that I secretly coveted. I profoundly appreciate the bravery it took for her to agree to care for our mother to give me the time and energy to complete this manuscript. For this, I will forever be in my sister's debt.

Matt Wolf-Meyer encouraged me to explore my narcolepsy as a scholar and autoethnographer before anyone else did. Erin Labbie, a graduate professor we both had while at Bowling Green State University, had alerted us to our mutual interest in researching sleep as a social practice. It has been a pleasure to follow his career and research since then. I also appreciate the thoughtful feedback and encouragement he offered on the book project and specific chapters.

Carl Lindahl is an exemplary researcher whose work deeply influenced my decision to model my interviews after the interviews I conducted as a part of the Surviving Katrina and Rita in Houston project. Following the Hurricane Katrina that flooded New Orleans, Carl Lindahl and Pat Jasper worked to develop the first large-scale effort to have survivors of these natural disasters interview each other to collect rich and personal accounts that generally covered three topics: their lives before the storm, their experience of the storm, and their new lives in the Greater Houston area. Participating in these interviews introduced me to the healing potential of such exchanges and to opportunities to write and publish my Katrina story alongside the stories of my interviewees. It also gave me, a reticent introvert, a rare opening to forge new connections in a city I had seemingly abandoned for college and graduate school. Carl's support helped turn my dreams of attaining a PhD into a reality.

Diana Bowen eagerly introduced me to communication studies when I was gearing up to apply to PhD programs. She discussed the overlap of cultural studies and communication before she shared that unlike many of the other humanities and social science degree programs I was considering, communication studies had a job market for its PhD holders. As I neared the end of my PhD program, we reconnected, and she offered to mentor me as I embarked on the many challenges that awaited me. Her exuberance and encouragement have helped me tremendously throughout this journey in academia.

J.W. Smith helped me address some of the turbulence I encountered while in the PhD program while also proving time and time again he was a resource graduate students could turn to outside of the decorum a classroom or office might impose. As a fellow Black disabled scholar, I appreciate his wisdom and example more than most. He introduced me to two others who I would like to thank and acknowledge here: Daryl Purdy and Jenny Nelson. I am deeply indebted to Daryl's fierce advocacy and willingness to fight for people with disabilities. Jenny's friendship and mentorship, as a fellow academic and neurological misfit, meant we were able to share parts of ourselves that we may have otherwise hidden away.

I would like to acknowledge how my interest in writing poetically, creatively, and performatively was inspired by the works of Ron Pelias and Phil Smith, who both skillfully blend the tools of poetry and research. I also want to express my appreciation for the support Julie-Ann Scott-Pollock and Craig Gingrich-Philbrook provided to some of my earlier performative writings. I would like to also express my admiration and appreciation for the creative juggernaut Darrel Alejandro Holnes, a friend and fellow Katrina interviewer.

Sarah Parsloe's feedback on my earlier drafts helped embolden a timidity that may have otherwise flourished. Her companionship as a fellow health communication scholar meant I was not truly alone, especially during our first years of that program. My dissertation committee, Lynn Harter, J.W. Smith, and Risa Whitson, have been courageous sources of inspiration and guidance during my time at Ohio University and beyond. My former advisor, William K. Rawlins, has done a masterful job at setting the beat for our ongoing jam session, and I am honored to be able to keep the music playing throughout the rest of my measures. I am truly grateful for countless ways he has continued to support my work while personifying compassion and eloquence. I would also like to thank Michael Butterworth and the Ohio University's School of Communication Studies for providing financial support for my many trips to and from Columbus, Ohio.

In 2019, I attended the National Communication Association's faculty development program that used to go by the name of the Hope Conference, because Hope University offered to host it for several years. They offer faculty who teach only undergraduates an opportunity to take mini seminars to reengage with scholarship or to explore approaches to research. This is where I had an opportunity to learn with Carolyn Ellis and the other colleagues who selected to explore autoethnography with her. Carolyn provided meticulous and thoughtful feedback on chapter 2 and a chapter that I decided to remove to publish in another venue. Catherine Squire's class on yoga and trauma triggered an ongoing transformation that is difficult to describe. I'll say that it is comprised of countless brushstrokes that pointed the way for me to rediscover the woman who fell in love with poetry and performance and was courageous enough to follow this siren. I would like to also express my profound gratitude for the full-throated praise, meticulous feedback, and enthusiastic encouragement my devoted husband and scholar, Josiah Rector, has provided me time and time again.

I want to recognize the informal and/or formal support I received from Zamzam Jama, Nadya Pittendrigh, Liane Tanguay, Kyoko Amano, Nate Hodges, Laura Ellingson, Andrew Baerg, Tony Adams, Jennifer Hawkins, Jeffrey R. Di Leo, Chance Glenn, Thomas Weller, Gerard J. Meskill, and

Julie Flygare. Lastly, I want to thank everyone at Lexington Press who helped bring this book to press. I really appreciate my initial editor Nicolette Amstutz and the assistance I received from Deja Ryland. I deeply appreciate the help and guidance Jessie Tepper provided through the manuscript preparation process. Susan Higgins is the proofreader, and Jessica McCleary is the production editor who wondrously transformed the manuscript into sleek and polished finished product.

Chapter 1

Exploring Communication about Narcolepsy

Having arrived a few minutes early I wait in my car until 11:00 a.m., which is when the meeting is scheduled to start. As usual, there are plenty of parking spaces beside the former industrial manufacturing building whose twenty-five pane windows now belonged to artists who rent mini art studios in the building. As I reach the sidewalk corner, I notice that an artist stuck giant stickers of pastel-colored cats sitting with their backs to us on the bricks—each time I come here something is different about the building, the space, the parking, or the nearby buildings. This place is alive like that. The restaurant, Strongwater Food and Spirits, is probably a big part of why. It proudly retains many of the architectural features from when it was once the headquarters for the sanitary porcelain manufacturing company that built the building in 1901. Upon entering, I look down at the “EBCO” encircled on the stone floor and start to wonder what the initials could mean. While unsuccessfully searchin for any word combinations I am greeted by an unfamiliar person—a cent Asian man with gratuitous facial hair who is donning the same trendy ar vibe I have come to expect here.

“Hi, I’m here for the meeting” I tell him while pointing to claim our d less room. His facial expression tells me he has no idea what I am ta about. So, I attempt an explanation, “Every month a narcolepsy support meets here,” pointing to rooms that likely used to be offices where the pants could see employees come and go through the large glass windo take up two walls.

“Oh, okay. Do you need anything?”

Reaching into my shoulder bag to get my pad folio I reply, “I n tape to put up a sign.”

“I think I can find it. So, others are coming? What type did you say?”

"It's a narcolepsy support group," I offer, and look around. While pointing to four tubes of florescent lightbulbs hanging from what might be a ten-foot ceiling, I ask, "Do you know anything about the lighting? Do any of these lights work?" I note that, "It's kinda weird for us to meet in such a dark area." The room where we usually meet is partially lit from two shade-less lamps and from the flood of light emanating from the windows in front of the building. Despite the bright teal accent wall, the candy-colored chairs, and all the light from a bright nearly cloudless day, the room feels dark because of all the dark features—the black walls, the high black ceiling, the dark paintings, the dark art deco buffet, the dark polished concrete floor, the dark finish on the wood that frames the windows, and the dark table which is the largest item in the little nook. Darkness tends to evoke sleep for me. This is why I have come to slightly loathe the trend of dim and dark eating establishments.

He starts to look around the room for a switch, and when he does not find one, he admits that he does not know what is going on with the lights. He aves to fetch the tape.

spot Noelle, the slim White woman, who wears her waist-length hair in se messy bun; she usually serves us and knows about the support group. the awkward exchange with her coworker, I appreciate her familiar e all the more. She brings me the tape and offers to bring me one of emade ginger ales. With two pieces of tape, I tape the paper onto the help newcomers find the meeting. The sign says, "Narcolepsy Not ink highlighter—which is all I could find in my bag. This phrase f Julie Flygare's campaign to help people with narcolepsy feel supported (Project Sleep, n.d.).

round, I notice that the artwork on the accent wall changed meeting. Beside the familiar large surrealist painting are that I move towards to inspect. Today there are four min- the other side of the wall, but I wonder what was there ized globe here last time? Or is it new too? Unable to , I abandon this worry. Perhaps I should have taken before brushing this idea away too. I head back to and pull out *The New Yorker* magazine but sud- uld look friendlier for newcomers. If someone ng, would they feel like they are distracting me y? Yet, for a person who dislikes waiting, this waiting usually means having a surplus of t could go wrong, are wrong, and might be ething I excel at.

lightly as I register my regret about the music this morning. Wondering who l phone to check the event posted on the support group's Facebook page. Two unfamiliar names and two familiar names indicated they would come. What happened? Did they all simply forget? Is 11:00 a.m. too early?

A couple enters the restaurant. I find myself creating a story about them and their whispered search for the support group meeting. Even as they sit at a table that is in my line of sight, I hesitantly imagine that they are going to wait to see if anyone else comes before deciding to join me. Again, this is an enormously unproductive line of thinking. Once I admit to myself that they were merely customers, I am relieved to find that the truth did not accompany a sting of rejection. Soon, another person comes into the restaurant, and this time I resist the urge to imagine that they are headed this way as they glide past the doorway. Eventually fifteen minutes have passed, and I am still here alone. A few more moments pass, and I am offered another ginger ale. I take it. When Noelle returns with it, she sympathizes with me and tells me that I am free to wait or leave. She also says that my drinks are on the house, filling me with genuine astonishment and gratitude before the posture of worry returns.

While playing Candy Crush, I finally admit to myself that the meeting is not going to happen today. However, I am not as disappointed as I was the first time it happened. Determined to make the most of this hour-plus trip to Columbus, I silence all the negative meanings I could take from this experience and instead choose to accept this trip and the account that emerges from it as an illustration of the unpredictable nature of both fieldwork and narcolepsy. Sitting in that darkly lit room, I start to toy with the idea of making this experience a more explicit part of the research narrative. Later, once I returned to my muted yellow hotel room, the seed of this idea matured into a decision to detail my account. I quickly scribble fieldnotes about the details of the non-meeting before the vivid memories of the morning faded away.

The story of sitting alone behind a sign that said, "Narcolepsy Not Alone" symbolized what I sought to capture in my research on people with narcolepsy—it illuminated the precise yet elusive absence and a requisite presence that connects individuals who are often too tired, too forgetful, too busy, or too sleepy to participate in aspects of everyday life. This pattern of disengagement is not exclusive to the specific condition of narcolepsy and immediately adjacent conditions. I suspect there are many conditions and support groups that leave group leaders similarly sitting alone wondering if anyone will come while nevertheless also empathizing with their inability to come. In many ways narcolepsy is a chronic health condition that creates predictable and unscheduled absences in a world that gives adults and children awards for simply showing up consistently. Like the little changes I found in each visit to Strongwater, as someone with narcolepsy it is incredibly hard to account for what is absent or what I missed due to sleepiness or naps. Alternatively, while the condition is an unambiguous absence, it is also much more than a list of missed opportunities, late arrivals, missed classes, canceled RSVPs, rainchecks for after-parties or incomplete projects. The subjective experience of living with narcolepsy also entails bizarre voyages into states few people know exist much less visit—the spaces between awake and sleep, between dreams and reality, between subject and object, between action and inaction. This book is an introduction to some of the places people with narcolepsy frequent and to the situations they find themselves in when sleepiness and other symptoms of narcolepsy appear. Readers should finish this book with an expanded ability to regard a sleepy or sleeping person in public or in another unexpected context with a greater measure of compassion, sympathy, and curiosity.

Many people regard sleep as an absence where meaningful life ends and an experience akin to death unfolds. In a 24/7 culture the trend is for people to sleep less and less to accomplish the ever-expanding list of things one can or must do (Crary, 2013). Another type of absence that narcolepsy creates is based on how the person with narcolepsy often is unable to fully participate in the way the absence is interpreted in the precise moment where someone sees the symptoms of narcolepsy. In the same way that I experienced the absent group members, people with narcolepsy who are not able to show up or are tardy often may leave others to make sense of the absence with little or no honest input from the absent party. The myriad challenges of communicating about narcolepsy often compound the social isolation narcolepsy imposes. I seek to fill in these absences by doing what the sleeping narcoleptic cannot do—that is, I will be the narcoleptic that actively shapes how their experience is understood with brutal honesty and situated nuance. In addition to shaping how the experiences of others with narcolepsy are understood, I am also interested in offering my story to the reader as I did for each of the people I interviewed. By using narratives extensively throughout this book, I am performing the exchange of stories central to how many people cope with having a disabling chronic condition. These exchanges unfold in an interview context that includes me sharing my story with my interviewee to invite them into the opportunity to make sense of our experiences together. This dialogic format seeks to spawn similar dialogues by inspiring further qualitative work on disability and rare disease communities.

Living with narcolepsy creates innumerable elusive absences in my life that writing allows me to access and research allows me to interrogate and shape. Instead of being satisfied with making sense of how others understand my narcolepsy post hoc or a priori, this book allows me to stand in the shoes of the other—usually the non-narcoleptic—to appreciate narcolepsy from multiple perspectives.

Contemporary medical treatment effectively manages the most debilitating aspects of narcolepsy, for most patients, and this should never be minimized or undermined. The value medical treatment of symptoms creates in the lives of people with narcolepsy is immeasurable. Yet patients' voices and experiences are largely absent from medical literature on narcolepsy as they are in many medical contexts. Particularly, since the invention of electroencephalography (EEG) and other tools for interrogating the patient's body, the use of patient narratives and self-reports has been less essential in diagnosing and treating sleep disorders (Kroker, 2007). The ricocheting line of an EEG tells sleep specialists what is and is not happening in the brain of someone with narcolepsy, which inadvertently minimizes the role of patient accounts in clinical encounters. The vulnerable and deeply disempowering symptoms of narcolepsy are too often relatively voiceless in both everyday life and medical contexts. Narrative medicine has long sought to repair the resulting chasm between the body and the voice of the patient (Kleinman, 1988). This book aims to carve a new path between the body and the narrative life by telling the stories of people with narcolepsy and adding thick description to existing medically accurate accounts of life with narcolepsy. The meaning of narcolepsy—that is the meaning of sleep, sleepiness, and the other symptoms of narcolepsy—is shaped by complex, interwoven interactions that are specific to individuals and the places they occur. By communicating about narcolepsy in the places where people with narcolepsy experience disabling symptoms, doctors and other support persons may better understand what narcolepsy means in the lives of those who live with it.

This chapter introduces narcolepsy and discusses the goals of this book, which are twofold: to create an account of narcolepsy that recognizes its unique absences, and to use the inspiration gleaned from performative writing to craft narratives that reveal how people with narcolepsy navigate everyday life. First, I will provide a detailed description of narcolepsy based on medical literature. Afterward it describes the rationale for this research and the main theoretical considerations informing this inquiry. Lastly, this chapter concludes with a summary of the chapters that follow.

By following the opening phenomenological narrative about narcolepsy with a medical approach to communicating about narcolepsy, I am highlighting the way considerations of genre like form and voice construct distinct portraits of narcolepsy. The narratives also draw attention to the nuances involved in how the body co-authors the one's story of life as one lives it (Charon, 2006). Like the opening narrative, the medical description is also a compelling illustration of narcolepsy that is essentially a type of story. Most of the medical story, which has the support and legitimacy of medical institutions and all the subsequent epistemological infrastructure that supports medicine, still re-inscribes the absences that narcolepsy creates by leaving the everyday lived experiences of those who live with the condition muted. And yet, this bleak and undermining impact of the medical story is something many people cling to upon diagnosis because often prior to learning of the medical language offered by sleep medicine, many feel like they have no words at all to communicate about living with a uniquely vulnerable condition.

A MEDICAL DESCRIPTION OF NARCOLEPSY

Approximately one in two thousand Americans have narcolepsy; in Japan, the rate is one in six hundred; and in Israel the rate is one in five hundred thousand (Siegel, 2000). To put the American rate into context, it is an incidence rate that is half that of multiple sclerosis, and it is about a quarter of the incidents of Parkinson's disease and five times the incidence rate of cystic fibrosis (Siegel, 2000). Narcolepsy typically develops when the patient is a teenager or in their twenties and can worsen at a later age (Dauvilliers et al., n.d.; Siegel, 2000). Often, diagnosis is delayed by an average of ten years because people with narcolepsy are frequently diagnosed with other conditions before seeing a sleep specialist and receiving the correct diagnosis (Kryger et al., 2002). Narcolepsy typically has a gradual onset, but the onset can be sudden or be due to other conditions (American Academy of Sleep Medicine, 2014). Unfamiliarity with the condition among health care providers contributes to the significant length of time that typically precedes diagnosis and subsequent treatment (Thorpy & Krieger, 2014). Narcolepsy is a neurological sleep disorder, and it is a lifelong chronic condition that is caused by an autoimmune response and therefore is an autoimmune condition that may accompany other autoimmune conditions (Dauvilliers et al., n.d.). Narcolepsy occurs in both sexes with a slight preponderance of males (American Academy of Sleep Medicine, 2014).

Narcolepsy is linked to neurological mechanisms that control sleep/wake cycles (Siegel, 2000). There are two main phases of sleep: REM sleep and non-REM sleep. REM stands for rapid eye movement, which is what happens when sleepers are dreaming. During REM sleep the brain's metabolism exceeds what happens when awake, and muscle tone is absent in legs and arms to not act out dreams (Siegel, 2000). Non-narcoleptics will spend approximately ninety minutes in non-REM sleep, a quiet phase of sleep when the brain is not consuming a lot of energy, before transitioning to REM sleep (Siegel, 2000). The EEG sleep tests that diagnose narcolepsy look for signs that the sleeper is skipping non-REM sleep and going directly to REM sleep in under fifteen minutes. The sleep tests for narcolepsy include the multiple sleep latency test (MSLT) which involves having a person take naps during the day while monitored by polysomnography. The MSLT looks for an average onset of sleep of under eight minutes. A spinal tap can also be used to confirm narcolepsy with cataplexy (Dauvilliers, 2007; Siegel, 2000). There are two types of narcolepsy: type 1 is otherwise known as narcolepsy *with* cataplexy, and type 2 is often called narcolepsy *without* cataplexy (American Academy of Sleep Medicine, 2014). In alignment with medical journals that discuss the two types, I will use the more familiar term *narcolepsy* to refer to both types, and where the type is relevant I will indicate *with cataplexy* or *without cataplexy* where appropriate.

Narcolepsy without Cataplexy (Type 2)

The primary symptom for narcolepsy without cataplexy, which hereafter will be referred to as narcolepsy, is excessive daytime sleepiness (EDS). EDS is the most severe symptom and is usually the reason patients seek medical attention (Dauvilliers, 2007). This most often is the first symptom to appear (Dauvilliers, 2007). Sleepiness can gradually increase in intensity or it can be without prodromal symptoms—the sudden onset of sleep without warning is called "sleep attacks" (American Academy of Sleep Medicine, 2014). The term *sleep attacks* has also been used to describe moments of sleepiness that may not result in sleep (Merritt et al., 1992). In his description of the epidemiological and clinical features of narcolepsy with cataplexy, Yves Dauvilliers (2007) describes EDS in these terms:

> Daytime sleepiness occurs daily, recurring typically at 2-h intervals, exacerbated during inactivity, with large variability between patients. Most of those sleep episodes are irresistible, of short duration and frequently associated with dreaming. . . . Severe sleepiness can also lead to unconscious microsleep episodes or lapses. (p. 338)

This description of EDS applies to both types of narcolepsy. There is ambiguity about the meaning of the term *sleep attack* and therefore it is rarely used in literature about narcolepsy. The third edition of the *International Classification of Sleep Disorders (ICSD-3),* published by the American Academy of Sleep Medicine, describes hypersomnolance, or daytime sleepiness, as the "inability to stay awake and alert during the major waking episodes of the day, resulting in periods of irrepressible need for sleep or unintended lapses into drowsiness or sleep" (American Academy of Sleep Medicine, 2014, p. 143). People with narcolepsy experience EDS, meaning that excessive sleepiness has occurred at least over a three-month period (American Academy of Sleep Medicine, 2014). The severity of sleepiness can vary, and sleepiness is more likely to occur in sedentary places, boring and monotonous situations, and might be accompanied by memory lapses, automatic behavior, drooping eyelids, blurred vision, or double vision (American Academy of Sleep Medicine, 2014). While other conditions may include EDS, nowhere does it appear more severe than in narcolepsy (Mayer et al., 2013).

Other common narcolepsy symptoms include sleep paralysis, hypnagogic hallucinations, epic dreams, and nocturnal sleep disruption (American Academy of Sleep Medicine, 2014). Sleep paralysis is when, upon waking or falling asleep, someone finds that they are unable to move. It is transient, meaning the ability to move returns after one or more minutes (American Academy of Sleep Medicine, 2014). The *ICSD-3* defines hypnogogic hallucinations as, "vivid dreamlike experiences occurring in the transition from wake to sleep. Typically, hypnogogic hallucinations have a multimodal or 'holistic' character, often combining visual, auditory and tactile phenomena" (American Academy of Sleep Medicine, 2014, p. 148). People with narcolepsy are more than twice as likely to be obese (American Academy of Sleep Medicine, 2014). Other common comorbidities include anxiety, fatigue, and other sleep abnormalities (American Academy of Sleep Medicine, 2014). People with narcolepsy have high rates of depression, with some studies reporting that over 50 percent of participants experienced this comorbidity (Won et al., 2014). Compared to non-narcoleptics, people with narcolepsy are two to four times more likely to develop psychiatric conditions (Flores et al., 2016).

Narcolepsy is treated with stimulant drugs to suppress the effects of daytime sleepiness; tricyclic antidepressants are often used to treat cataplexy; and hydroxybutyrate and pitolisant (Wakix) has been used to treat both symptoms (Dauvilliers et al., n.d.; Meskill et al., 2021). Sodium oxybate (Xyrem and Lumryz) and calcium, magnesium, potassium, and sodium oxybates (Xywav) are also used to treat disrupted nighttime sleep and alleviate EDS and cataplexy. There are some cognitive behavioral therapy approaches to treatment, but guidelines for these approaches still need to be developed (Marín Agudelo et al., 2014). Since narcolepsy recently was declared an autoimmune condition, there currently are no FDA-approved immunotherapy options for treatment but this is an area where researchers are laying the foundation for new medicines and treatments.

In 2009, during the influenza pandemic, a vaccine for H1N1 was developed and distributed in various countries in Europe. Clinicians in Finland and Sweden noticed an increase in the incidents of narcolepsy and identified a relationship between the increase and vaccinations for the influenza vaccine in patients in England, Ireland, France, and Norway (American Academy of Sleep Medicine, 2014; Barker & Snape, 2014). As of 2015, over two hundred children and adults in Europe developed narcolepsy as a result of the Pandemrix vaccination (Lundgren, 2015).

Narcolepsy with Cataplexy (Type 1)

Narcolepsy with cataplexy represents a subset of the population of people with narcolepsy and is generally regarded as more severe. Although these numbers will vary widely from one study to the next, the American Academy of Sleep Medicine (2014) estimated that narcolepsy with cataplexy counts for approximately 15 to 25 percent of the population of people with narcolepsy. Significantly more is known about the physiopathology of this form of narcolepsy because the gene for this type of narcolepsy has been identified in dogs, meaning that researchers are able to give a dog narcolepsy with cataplexy to study the neurological mechanisms at work (Siegel, 2000). Narcolepsy with cataplexy is caused by a marked reduction of hypocretin, a chemical created in the hypothalamus and involved in sustaining alertness and controlling when REM sleep occurs (American Academy of Sleep Medicine, 2014). People may be diagnosed with type 1 narcolepsy even though they do not have cataplexy because the definitive trait for this form of narcolepsy is decreased hypocretin (American Academy of Sleep Medicine, 2014).

People diagnosed with narcolepsy with cataplexy also experience the symptoms of narcolepsy without cataplexy. Cataplexy is an intriguing example of how thoughts affect neurological function (Krahn et al., 2005). It is defined as the sudden loss of bilateral muscle tone in response to a strong emotion, which may be referred to as an emotional trigger (American Academy of Sleep Medicine, 2014). Cataplexy can typically look like involuntary eye closure, knee weakness, slurred speech, inability to hear, head droop, jaw slacking, facial weakness, or the total loss of muscle tone throughout the body (Krahn et al., 2005). These cataplexy episodes, or attacks, may last a few seconds or a few minutes during which consciousness is clear, memory is uninterrupted, and breathing is normal (American Academy of Sleep Medicine, 2014). Delays in diagnosis are connected to patients' difficulty describing the experience and to the way cataplexy happens only with specific triggers; therefore, it may remain too elusive for doctors to observe it during a brief office visit (Won et al., 2014). Women are more likely to develop cataplexy than men (Won et al., 2014). The decreased muscle tone of cataplexy is similar to the decrease in muscle tone during REM sleep (Krahn et al., 2005). More than any other emotion, laughter is the most likely trigger of cataplexy; other positive emotions may also be a trigger such as hearing a joke, feeling excited, feeling elated, remembering a happy moment, or experiencing an unspecified emotional event (Krahn et al., 2005). The frequency of cataplexy can range from less than once a month to more than twenty attacks a day (American Academy of Sleep Medicine, 2014).

RATIONALE FOR RESEARCHING EVERYDAY LIFE WITH NARCOLEPSY

The story of showing up to a narcolepsy support group meeting to find that no one came and the detailed medical description of narcolepsy are told from two different epistemologies and therefore both achieve distinct forms of knowledge creation. The story that opens the chapter relies on my subjective experience, embedded meanings, material resources, and metaphor. It is an emplaced story that represents a singular perspective that is unique to my experience. Conversely, the medical description of narcolepsy is an intricate amalgamation of information and research about a pathology that aims to be void of feelings and "bias" in accordance with a positivist paradigm. Medical and scientific language about narcolepsy provides a great deal of legitimacy and validation for people with narcolepsy, which is a privilege not afforded to many people with chronic fatigue syndrome or other syndromes since the designation "syndrome" indicates the absence of medical legitimacy (Japp & Japp, 2005, p. 114). Yet, however empowering it may seem, medical jargon about sleep disorders often fails to help people with narcolepsy accomplish the work of communicating about their condition to family, friends, coworkers, and employers (Young, 2013). Nor does it help make everyone with narcolepsy feel empowered to live in a world where sleep is often devalued and sleepiness is easily misunderstood. Medical language also fails to imagine or anticipate how culture, race, and power may influence how symptoms are experienced or are understood.

In Susan Wendell's (1996) book, *The Rejected Body,* she describes how the authority of medicine over people's ability to communicate about their own bodies is a type of epistemic invalidation because medicine can undermine our confidence in our ability to know our own bodies in the space between the words used to describe personal experiences and the words used in medical descriptions (p. 122). Before being diagnosed with narcolepsy, many of my participants, and myself included, were told, "There's nothing wrong with you," or were misdiagnosed, compelling a choice between distrusting our own knowledge about our bodies or distrusting the judgment of a medical professional. Once diagnosed, however, people with narcolepsy are released from epistemic invalidation.

The medical jargon used to describe narcolepsy above was created to accomplish the goals of researchers and doctors. According to Matt Wolf-Meyer (2012), a medical anthropologist and the author of *Slumbering Masses,* medical interest in treating narcolepsy was motivated by an impulse to defend patients against dominant understandings of narcoleptics as being "willfully lazy" (p. 76). Sleep medicine asserted that, rather than being a choice, narcolepsy occurs because of a problem of the nervous system. However, sleep medicine is not without cultural biases. Rather, the way meanings of sleep, sleepiness, and alertness have evolved in that domain reflect the sociohistorical biases of the men who were influential in establishing the ideas, the language, and the technological tools of sleep medicine (Wolf-Meyer, 2012). According to Wolf-Meyer (2012):

> Restless legs syndrome, narcolepsy, and REM behavior disorder are all problematic at the turn of the twenty-first century because of what they index *socially*. . . . and variation from sleep's consolidation and hegemony is not simply resistance but also disorder. (p. 77)

In embracing medical language about sleep, people with narcolepsy also embrace the underlying logic it presents: which is that the malleability of sleep must be put in alignment with spatiotemporal rhythms of society by using medicine instead of expecting society to become more malleable to better accommodate irrepressible sleepiness (Wolf-Meyer, 2012). In other words, sleep medicine has protected narcolepsy from moral degradation, but in accepting this assistance, they are also agreeing to value and understand sleep primarily based on socially constructed norms of sleep medicine.

Perhaps there is a third way forward? Are there ways to communicate about narcolepsy that are not imposed by intransigent institutional jargon? Is there a way to communicate about narcolepsy that uses medical knowledge, personal narrative, and metaphor without invalidating or delegitimizing these epistemologies? In exploring how people with narcolepsy understand narcolepsy, I resist rendering them, once again, as passive patients by putting the subjective experiences of narcolepsy in conversation with the medical language of narcolepsy. This book wants both to be a bridge and build a bridge between these two ways of knowing about narcolepsy, while making a substantive contribution to the social and cultural study of sleep.

Representation is central to the types of knowledge that may be produced. Therefore, I sought to design a research project that created representations of narcolepsy that would help to fill in many of the holes that more empirical research on the topic has created while also protecting participants by using pseudonyms and other measures discussed in the appendix. Accordingly, the central problem this book seeks to address is the question of what narcolepsy means to the people who live with it. How do they experience the absences? Or how does it feel to have found the right job, spouse, or friend? Who understands and supports them? What does it mean to have narcolepsy symptoms while in specific places?

Lastly, I would like to address some of the terms used in discussions of narcolepsy. The word *narcolepsy* means sleep seizure (Wolf-Meyer, 2012).

While narcolepsy has at times been called an *illness* or a *disease,* people who have it and those who work with them tend to call narcolepsy a *condition* or a *sleep disorder*. Although it is considered a type of chronic illness, the term *illness* refers to an individual's perceptions of their symptoms and how they are experienced by family members and themselves (Falvo, 2009). Additionally, while the term *disease* refers to changes in the structure or function of a body, this term is rarely if ever used in contemporary discussions of narcolepsy (Falvo, 2009).

Theorizing Narcolepsy as a Hidden Disability

People with disabilities are the largest minority group in the United States, and it is a group that anyone can join with little notice or choice in the matter because everyone is vulnerable to debility (Baglieri et al., 2011). People who have different embodiments—disfigurement, medical conditions, etc.—have been the subject of poking, prodding, disciplining, distrust, and dismissal throughout history. Until recent years, people did not identify with the label "disabled"; rather it was crudely assigned to a person to designate a devalued social status (Goffman, 2006, p. 141). Ervin Goffman (2006) was one of the earliest researchers to study the social process of stigmatizing in *Stigma: Notes on the Management of Spoiled Identity,* and, in some ways, he was a proto-disability studies scholar. Goffman's work spoke to the experience of navigating a world that saw people with disabilities as less than. According to Rosemarie Garland-Thomson (2014), in her biographical essay, "The story of my work: How I became disabled," the U.S. civil rights movement and the Black Power movement provided a framework for people who were labeled as inferior and wrong—the disabled—to speak back to "this accusation of wrongness" (para. 9). Lennard Davis (2006) breaks the disability movement into two waves: in the first wave, in the 1970s and 1980s, people were in solidarity against the oppressive regime of ableism. In the second wave of the 1990s, the solidarity was fractured and the movement was plagued with internal conflict (p. 231). In both waves the goal was to put an end to how medical language characterized disability and replace it with a language that recognized the social process of putting restrictions and limitations on what and how people accomplished things in everyday life (Davis, 2006).

The social model of disability was created to address how restrictions put on people with disabilities originate in social attitudes and structures and not with the physical state of a particular embodiment (Shakespeare, 2006). The social model challenges the legitimacy and the tyranny of the medical model of disability, which was used by nonmedical professionals and nondisabled people to justify denying privileges, assistance, and voices to people labeled disabled, incompetent, feeble, mad, and the like. Wielding the social model of disability, the disability rights movement and the disability pride movement brought about the passage of the Americans with Disabilities Act in 1990, while also raising the profile of people with disabilities in various aspects of culture and everyday life.

Disability studies also took root in academia during this period. In 1982, the *Disability and Chronic Disease Newsletter* was founded and eventually became *Disability Studies Quarterly,* a major source of interdisciplinary research on the topic of disability (Baglieri et al., 2011). In 1986, the Society for Disability Studies (SDS) was created, and this was a significant resource for creating community and legitimacy as an area of study. The social science core of disability studies scholarship was soon joined by humanities-based scholars who joined SDS and contributed to understanding disability as historians and cultural critics (Garland-Thomson, 2014). Humanities scholars brought a focus on narrative, aesthetics, and representation to the discussion of the social construction of disability. Prior to the 1990s, educators relied on the medical model, but after several conferences that focused on the intersection of education and disability, researchers and educators began to work on addressing the ways that education can approach disability in new ways, and this ongoing effort is called Disability Studies in Education (Baglieri et al., 2011). Currently, there are numerous opportunities in various sectors of society for disability studies scholars and activists to continue to transform the way disability is represented, treated, and constructed.

Disability and Identity

Identity is a complex and contentious issue within disability studies. While the disability pride movement and its various offshoots encourage people to claim their disability and to find community in being a person with a disability, there are many writers who have developed different positions on the issue. Garland-Thomson (2014), who was born with a limb difference, embraced disability as an identity because feminism taught her to be critical of messages that she was less than or inferior. In other words, feminism introduced her to positive identity politics and demonstrated how embracing a marginalized identity could serve academic and activist objectives. Similarly, Nick Walker, a leading voice in the neurodiversity movement, embraces autism as an identity category, contending that as a minority group, "people with disabilities" does not compute. He points out in the case of race and sexuality we say, "she's black" or "she's a lesbian" (Walker, 2013, para. 18). Yet, as he further explains:

> If we use phrases like "person with Autism," or "she has Autism," or "families affected by Autism," we're using the language of the pathology paradigm—language that implicitly accepts and reinforces the assumption that Autism is intrinsically a problem, a Something-Wrong-With-You. (Walker, 2013, para. 19)

Walker enthusiastically embraces his autism and wants to be called autistic. To him, people-first language legitimizes the devaluation of difference when disability activists and people with disabilities should be encouraged to value their unique embodiment. Meanwhile, Davis (2006) argues that if disability is socially constructed and therefore is an unstable category, then instead of reifying the social construction of disability, scholars should try to move beyond identity politics and amplify the instability of the category).

Alternatively, people living with disabling physical pain may chafe at the suggestion that they should embrace their disability as an identity. This would be tantamount to embracing their bodily pain. Narcolepsy is at the intersection of conditions that impose unenviable experiences that are not easily embraced and neurodiversity conditions that challenge conceptions of normal brains. On good days, I embrace narcolepsy as a neurodiversity condition, but then there are rare days when I chafed at unplanned naps and the undone work they often create. The nature of narcolepsy requires a stance towards disability that is flexible and can appreciate the diverse stances people with narcolepsy may take towards issues of disability and identity. I use both person first language (e.g., person with narcolepsy) and identity language (e.g., narcoleptic) in recognition of the multiple stances people with narcolepsy may take towards the topic of identity language.

Rather than focusing on identity, many people who research disabilities are more interested in researching and theorizing around the choice to "pass" as able-bodied or the choice to identify as disabled through disclosure, requesting accommodations, or everyday practices (Carey, 2013; Cox, 2013; Samuels, 2015; Scott, 2015; Valeras, 2010). While this project began as an inquiry into the ways people with narcolepsy navigate these types of issues, it became clear at an early stage that, as Walker (2013) suggests, it is essential to recognize language that implies that something is wrong with human variation. To access the lived realities of people with narcolepsy, I had to critique and dismiss ideas that could potentially lead to replicating the alienation created by medical discourses on narcolepsy.

Narcolepsy and Place

In approaching a condition like narcolepsy, I sought to interrogate assumptions about the relationship between visibility, knowledge, and disability. The expectation that all disabilities be translated into objective knowledge is not a neutral appeal—a body's ability to produce knowledge via measurements, tests, exercises, and observation occurs in sociohistorical cultural landscapes (Chesler, 2005; Haraway, 1999; Silberman, 2016). In other words, must a researcher seek out bodies that have been medically diagnosed and therefore seen under the right conditions by the right people to reflect the right medical constructs? Alternatively, resisting acquiescence to social, personal, and political forces that obfuscate and distort bodies into silence also has troublesome implications. That is, to render a person in a way that lifts them into an abstracted argument about the way bodies are reflections of discourse enacts a different type of misrepresentation. Even so, I would like to argue that this is a false dilemma. Knowledge production about disabilities does not need to choose between the language of biomedical sciences and the language of the humanities or social sciences. Many researchers seek to develop descriptions of disability in situ—amidst the experiences of everyday life (Butler & Derrett, 2014; Jaeger, Röjvik, & Berglund, 2015; Wolf-Meyer, 2014). Such work labors to *see* disabilities on their own terms—to grasp the interactions between bodies and their physical and social environment requires grappling with the dilemmas of such an attempt.

An uncritical reliance on medical definitions to validate and to name impairments naturalizes pathologies. Wendell (1996) claims that the social and cognitive authority of medical descriptions of the body validates and invalidates how society supports or fails to support how individuals experience their bodies and selves. The consequence of investing tremendously into medical authority, according to Wendell (1996), is that it legitimates the treatment of people differently based on perceptions of social and cognitive authority—compounding the vulnerability of people who are poor, disabled, female, and/or non-White individuals.

As a researcher who identifies as having a neurological disability, it was imperative for me to grapple with the implications of researching my own condition. A specific diagnostic category is neither a neutral designator nor an apolitical object of investigation. By choosing to delineate an area of investigation along diagnostic lines as a researcher, there was also a concomitant choice to critically engage the institutions, the languages, and the procedures that have brought diagnostic criteria into existence, along with the discrete and diffused benefits of their deployment. Lastly, advocates for neurodiversity argue that individuals should have access to language that describes their constellation of mental processes without subjecting oneself to a pathology that often involves material and social consequences (Baker, 2011; Walker, 2013). If hidden disabilities are not sufficiently described by a list of pathologies—that is, autism, Parkinson's disease, post traumatic brain injury, bipolar disorder—then what is a hidden disability?

To approach hidden disability in a way that encourages language about the specific context, I have defined disability in similar terms to the World Health Organization (WHO). WHO defines disability as "the interaction between individuals with a health condition (e.g. cerebral palsy, Down syndrome, and depression) and personal and environmental factors (e.g. negative attitudes, inaccessible transportation and public buildings, and limited social supports)" (World Health Organization & World Bank, 2011, p. 4). Note that the key word here is *interaction.* This way of defining disability minimizes tendencies to judge ability and disability in a more cursory manner. In the definition of disability put forth by WHO, environmental factors refer to things that can either be a facilitator or a barrier. Environmental factors include products and technology; natural and built environments; support and relationships; attitudes; services, systems, and policies. These contextual factors interact with a person with a health condition in a way that creates a disability or enables the individual. Personal factors reference things like motivation and self-esteem that influence how much a person participates in society (World Health Organization & World Bank, 2011), while also including factors such as, "gender, race, education, occupation, and hard-to-quantify human factors such as past personal experiences, individual temperament, and other intrinsic characteristics such as state of mind" (Falvo, 2009, p. 4). This definition, and the International Classification of Functioning and Disability it draws on, turns disability into a continuum and abandons the tendency to regard it as a category. By looking at how narcolepsy interacts with contextual factors of a specific place, one can approach narcolepsy as a disability without imposing that label onto participants. This definition of disability also encourages an investigation of the role of place in the everyday life of people with narcolepsy.

Like the WHO definition of disability, hidden disabilities are about an interaction between bodies and place. By not defining hidden disabilities by the existence of a diagnostic category, we can focus on the interaction of disability—bodies in social contexts and physical spaces. It is this willingness to define disability as a site of interaction that allows researchers to approach these interactions as a source of heuristic insight. Moreover, it also allows researchers an ability to work in a way that is attuned to, "meanings that are masked, camouflaged, indirect, embedded, or hidden in context" (Conquergood, 2002, p. 146). For the motivating issues behind an in-situ approach to hidden disabilities are the many intricacies of how knowledge processes create places where some disabilities are self-evident while others are not.

To create a space for representations of hidden disabilities that disrupts unexamined assumptions about knowledge and visibility, I will define *hidden disability* using a specific disability context. A *hidden disability* is an impairment that occurs in specific contexts and spaces that impinge on an individual's ability to fulfill social roles and responsibilities. Take for example, narcolepsy is a neurological condition and it affects nearly all aspects of a patient's life. Accordingly, the pathology of attention deficit hyperactivity disorder (ADHD) and narcolepsy may seem quite different at face-value, but in a specific context the disability may be identical, if only for a moment. This is because excessive daytime sleepiness may affect a person's ability to focus. Therefore, a student with narcolepsy and a student with ADHD might both be at a disadvantage if they are in the back of the classroom, or near windows and doors that offer an endless parade of potential distractions. These dissimilar pathologies can yield similar experiences of disability (Falvo, 2009; Garland-Thomson, 2011). As a result, teachers, pedagogies, texts, activities, spaces, and interactions that expect these students to have an implicit capacity for attention and focus may similarly disable both students. In other words, context may be more significant than nuances of pathology.

Hidden disabilities can be hidden at multiple levels of interaction. Interpersonal communication and/or nonverbal communication can hide a disability; but more importantly, systems of organization and modes of interrogation may directly or indirectly hide persons and their differences. To call a condition or disability hidden is to situate it within a context that conceals a phenomenon. And it is this attention to context that unites all lived experiences for they all retain a potential for concealment. In other words, hidden disability, as a category, includes more apparent—physical—disabilities because in the right context they too may be concealed.

Contexts that hide how bodies differ may entail a set of tendencies, social positions, systems of thought, and pragmatic constraints. Taken together, these overlapping contexts may collude in obfuscating significant dimensions of human experience. Contexts that hide difference and deny the possibility of difference create the ontological experience of being hidden. As a person with narcolepsy, I exist within these interlaced contexts and therefore have access to interpretive frameworks that inform how I write about and see other people with narcolepsy. In my work, I seek to orchestrate a presentation of narcolepsy that situates it within everyday attunements and among the accumulated sensitivities that a life of performing a hidden disability makes possible. Accordingly, I write about such matters while also attending to the shifts between showing, knowing, and learning that are incumbent to this medium of exposition.

Misfitting as Lens

Western society once slept in configurations and patterns different from what is now observed. According to Roger Ekirch's (2006) award-winning research on sleep of pre-industrial England, their pattern was to go to sleep and to awake for a spell before returning to slumber. Wolf-Meyer (2012) claims that the current pattern of Americans sleeping in a consolidated block of time is a social norm that emerged with the help of medical dictates that claimed this to be optimal and natural. Sleep is a type of spatiotemporal social formation because it regulates and coordinates individuals and society (Wolf-Meyer, 2012). Normative spatiotemporal regimes occur at the level of individuals, organizations, populations, or across a society (Wolf-Meyer, 2012). For many people with sleep disorders, medication is a way of controlling an individual's body in relationship to the spatiotemporal expectations of everyday life (Wolf-Meyer, 2012).

The Americans with Disabilities Act has made significant advances since it passed in 1990; however, it has failed to integrate people with an array of impairments into economic and social life. This failure invites new and innovative projects that examine the barriers that keep people with disabilities unemployed and underemployed (Riviera Drew, 2015). My investigations of living with narcolepsy unite the humanities' contributions to disability studies with the knowledge production mechanisms of qualitative research to examine hidden disability as an enactment that is enmeshed within numerous dilemmas of representation. Moreover, hidden disabilities, like any other type of disability, are an instance of what Rosemarie Garland-Thomson (2011) calls misfitting. Misfits are bodies that must operate within environments that were built to fit a different type of body. Misfitting occurs, "when world fails flesh in the environment one encounters" (Garland-Thomson, 2011, p. 600). Facets of these environments include social, physical, geographical, and temporal placements. Misfits develop and deploy a range of strategies and capacities for coping with the misfit, and these responses to misfitting become the area of focus and not the intricacies of the embodiment or condition (Garland-Thomson, 2011).

I would like to extend Garland-Thomson's (2011) conception of misfitting to explicitly include the whole body—its brain, cognitive functions, emotions, and memories—that can either fit or misfit. Hidden disabilities—neurological conditions, psychological conditions, sensory conditions, immunological conditions, and others—are too often left out of discussions of how built environments may enable some bodies while disabling others (Baker, 2011; Dokumaci, 2014; Silberman, 2016). The concept of misfits is useful for hidden disability studies because it shirks off the less than useful attention to social/environmental deficits as well as the equally unproductive attention to impairments and deficits. Accordingly, the goal of *Asleep Anywhere* is to articulate how people with narcolepsy enact various strategies and abilities for dealing with the incongruencies between ability and place.

OVERVIEW OF CHAPTERS

In chapter 2, I use autoethnography to reflect on my journey with narcolepsy by sharing vignettes about being narcoleptic in specific places. This chapter recounts growing up Black around White children, my prediagnosis recollections of dealing with narcolepsy symptoms, dealing with narcolepsy during years of being uninsured, and during my PhD program prior to embarking on the research this book details. Each story reveals intimate details about what narcolepsy is and how my experience as is intertwined with my identity as a Black female.

Chapter 3 is an account of my time with Penny, who is married and is twenty-nine years old, and a newly diagnosed White woman with narcolepsy with cataplexy, who was previously diagnosed with ADHD, anxiety, and depression. When she began to fall asleep during the day while on stimulants for ADHD, her doctor suspected that Penny may have a sleep disorder. Penny chose to tell me more about her experience of having narcolepsy at work as an elementary school's speech pathologist, which is why I conducted her second interview in her classroom. Her stories of working with narcolepsy, one semester undiagnosed and one semester diagnosed, highlight four dimensions of experiencing narcolepsy at work: the presence of onlookers should one become sleepy or take a nap; the difficulty of working with sleepiness; inattention and other impairments; and the inflexible and flexible dimensions of the work environment.

Chapter 4 voices Elaine's narrative and illustrates what it means to have narcolepsy at home. I conducted only one interview with her, during which I asked about her home and saw that her account of having narcolepsy entails two distinct stories. One story involves working while narcoleptic, and the other is the story of being a mother of three young children while figuring out what narcolepsy means for her life and her family. This chapter will focus on the latter story but also recognizes that her understanding of what her home affords is based on comparisons to what her work affords. For Elaine, experiencing narcolepsy at home involves moments of fulfillment and moments of discontent with herself and others. For many of the people I interviewed, home was a site of multiple tensions; therefore, I also explore the stories of being home with narcolepsy from other support group members.

Chapter 5 focuses on the story of Sable, who gave up driving over a decade ago because of narcolepsy and multiple sclerosis. Sable is White and lives with her husband and receives disability retirement payments. Her diagnosis story details what it was like to talk about narcolepsy before popular culture depictions started to shape preconceptions about the condition. Sable described why she continued to drive despite her crashes and her uncontrolled cataplexy. Before giving up driving, Sable experienced conflicting feelings about driving with narcolepsy. Sable's ambivalence ended when the issue of immobility was resolved with the help of a coworker and a supportive husband.

Chapter 6 follows the story of Cynthia, who is an African American woman with narcolepsy that works for her family's funeral home. Cynthia wanted her second interview to be conducted at the ballet studio she attends. Her story highlights the struggle to manage medication side effects and the common comorbidity of depression. When dancing, her narcolepsy is backgrounded, and she feels unimpeded by it in this arena. Other interviewees highlighted the way they cherish being physically active by skateboarding or wind surfing. This chapter ends with my story of going to *The Wonderful Wizard of Oz* ballet where Cynthia danced as the Lion. I reflect on the story in terms of how it connects to my journey, while also discussing how the original story of *The Wonderful Wizard of Oz* highlighted the social construction of disability.

Chapter 7 reflects on some of the lessons learned about communicating about narcolepsy before returning to the questions that guided my time in the support group. In the discussion on the meanings of narcolepsy, the social construction of reality is used to facilitate a more sophisticated understanding of how narcolepsy may come to mean different things to different people. This chapter revisits many of the concepts from disability studies and to reiterate how messages about narcolepsy participate in producing enabling or disabling environments. The chapter closes with an exploration of how the narratives about narcolepsy presented here help with imagining a world where people like myself and my participants are better understood and are offered more options to sleep anywhere when navigating everyday life.

The appendix details the methodological dimensions of this exploration of narcolepsy and place. It includes a description of the history of the support group and my initial efforts to participate in meetings before the interviews could begin. The research influences and the interview process are explored along with the demographics of the group of people who participated in this research. The member check processes are discussed along with a few updates on the group since leaving Ohio. In the next chapter I narrate further some of my own experiences of living with narcolepsy.

Chapter 2

An Autoethnography on Being Black and/or Sleepy in the Right and Wrong Places

My experiences of hiding or revealing narcolepsy can be analyzed in relationship to the ways place is constructed through overlapping, complex, and contradictory messages. My immense reticence about sharing my life with this condition is accompanied by a meek bravery that builds on the many lessons I have learned from hearing the stories of other women with rare and not so rare disabilities (Bailey, 2017; Brown, 2019; Cohen, 2015; Defenbaugh, 2011; Dokumaci, 2014; Garland-Thomson, 2014; Grealy, 2016; Kafer, 2013; O'Rourke, 2022; Schalk, 2022; Scott, 2015; Tillman, 1996; Watkins, 2017; Wendell, 1996). In this chapter I use autoethnography to show that hidden disabilities like narcolepsy exist in places that may obscure how bodies may differ from one another. In other places these same disabilities may be perceived, acknowledged, and/or understood differently. In some contexts, sleepiness and/or sleep is benign, and in others it has dramatic consequences. As an autoethnographer, my racialized, gendered, neurodiverse body is continually entangled in the phenomenology of particular places (Pink, 2015). The significance of Blackness and narcolepsy is bound up to the places where they co-exist together.

To move into this mode of self-reflection and recollection, I have relied on models to guide the way. Rachel Alicia Griffin (2012) observed that in articulating her anger through writing a Black feminist autoethnography, she sought to do the exact thing that Black women are "discursively disciplined not to do" (p. 139). Various life experiences around disclosing narcolepsy have similarly discursively disciplined me to be overly cautious about disclosing narcolepsy and what it entails. My hesitant willingness to reveal the intricacies of sleepiness is a testimony to my belief in myself—my virtuosity, confidence, and resilience—in the face of a racist, sexist, and ableist world.

Yet, it would be naïve to breeze past the ways such an identity—Black, female, and neurodivergent—may be an uncomfortable fit within much of academia (Bailey, 2017). These incongruities are of particular interest here because they are sites of ongoing struggle. As discussed in chapter 1, the concept of a *misfit* describes encounters where the "world fails flesh in the environment one encounters" (Garland-Thomson, 2011, p. 600). Responses to misfitting—the new strategies and/or the coping practices a person pursues—may become the subject of analysis and therefore autoethnography is an opportunity to reflect on experiences of misfitting as opposed to focusing primarily on the susceptible embodiment, the pathology, the missing limb, the deafness, etc. Accordingly, this autoethnography seeks to reimagine ways of communicating about narcolepsy and Blackness by returning to the sites of misfitting and fitting to examine how someone adjusts and copes with being in a place that may not match one's embodiment or neurology.

The places people with narcolepsy occupy are tainted with the recognition that sleep, and sleepiness, may communicate unintended messages to people who observe and/or learn about such soporific departures. The stigma that often accompanies narcolepsy also relies on the uncritical dismissal of nonaction as lacking moral value (Kapella et al., 2015; Merritt, 2004; Price, 2021). The action and agency in writing about the lived experience of narcolepsy allows me to assert that despite the seeming lack of action inherent in the symptoms of narcolepsy, there is a lexicon of action, doing, and being folded between the poles of deep sleep and wakefulness. Communication persists in these spaces where bodies and intentional action are circumscribed by illness and disability. After all, as many contend, in enveloping contexts of meaning assignment people cannot not communicate (Watzlawick et al., 2014). The sleeping narcoleptic communicates despite living in a world that often does not listen to what they say. By accessing the relationship between place and narcolepsy, I am giving voice to the many ways meaning is woven into the silent syncope of narcolepsy symptoms.

I am not the same person who embarked on this project several years ago. Since then, I lost about thirty pounds and gained maybe twenty pounds and put a beloved pet to rest. I also accepted a tenure track position and jumped the broom. I have also reversed a horrid habit of collecting books that are almost never opened. The most dramatic transformation started when I discovered that many of my emotions were locked away many years ago, and in the following pages I recount some of the moments between being a child and becoming a professor that encouraged me to nurture distrust widely, to smother my feelings, and to hide my narcolepsy. Although this chapter's focus is squarely on my relationship with narcolepsy and the places symptoms emerge, know that this is but a small sliver of a rich, complex life. Ron Pelias's (2019) concept of a disrupted self allows autoethnographers to return to the site of a disruption to forge a narrative that might mute the chaos and rot that might otherwise reign unabated. In short, the shame, fear, and self-loathing that bubble up amid the disruptions narcolepsy created are moments that seek to give voice to those who are similarly trapped in layers of lessons that counsel to distrust, to be quiet, to disappear.

"IT'S TIME TO WAKE UP"

Houston 1990. "We're here. It's time to wake up," my dad announces as we pull into the driveway of a large two-story house that my parents bought. It's moving day.

This is the end of the seemingly endless drive from our previous mottled white brick home tucked in an area west of New Orleans. On the new house, the garage and square columns are cream, and the bricks are a rusty red. The smell of the new paint greets us inside. I recall how our seats in the van were first come, first serve, and imagine the policy for selecting a bedroom is probably also going to be first come, first serve. My sprint past my sisters telegraphs my thoughts. I aim to find the room with the window above the front door. As I turn the corner into the empty room I yell, "Mine! This room is mine!"

One sister runs past it to claim the next one but walks back adding, "I wanted that room."

Oh, the joys of being the oldest sibling. Her room has the walk-in closet. Something that I never really coveted until I lived in apartments that lacked them of course. That is much later. Right now, I am a nine-year-old girl in a house that smells of newness. After we are settled on the fact that the twins are sharing the room in the back, I return downstairs. The exploration of our new home can finally commence.

As I spot the backyard, I exclaim, "Look someone left the door open," as I start to run towards the lush green expanse. Of course, no one left the door open. My body slams against the crystal clean sliding glass door before flying backwards onto the floor.

First there is only silence.

Someone squeaks out a somewhat sincere, "Are you okay?"

Once I sit up and say, "Yeah," the room erupts in uncontrollable laughter. I am embarrassed like never before and yet I see the joke. Who does something like that? For years and decades, they laugh at my mistake. This is a story my sisters will never let me forget.

Third grade. Sitting on the floor with the rest of the kids. The teacher taps me on the shoulder and says, "Get more sleep at home." I do not know what she is talking about. I get plenty of sleep. I don't even remember falling asleep in class.

Fourth grade. I stay up past my bedtime drawing and coloring the book I wrote for my language arts class. The assignment was to write a book and I had been nurturing for some time a seed of an idea. This was the year I had begun experimenting with my hair occasionally. Even if it simply meant curling my bangs. The hairspray and a curling iron never seem to be enough to replicate what I saw in the *Ebony* or *Jet* magazines. I finally want to do something more than pushing my hair back into a ponytail. This yearning gave me an outline of a wish that I explored with my words and drawings. Christina, a Black girl like myself but a few years older, ends up going to the J.W. Watts beauty salon to get several makeovers only to inevitably discover her true self when she realizes she does not need the help of others to decide what she likes and how she should wear her hair. After Mrs. Watts reads the books we all wrote, she asks me to read my story to the class. She beams with pride. I'll never forget how my mouth felt like balls of cotton from reading my whole story aloud. I rarely said much in class, on the school bus, or at lunch while my peers seemed to talk endlessly in these spaces. No one else was given this opportunity to read aloud. Since then I nurtured a love of writing and began to turn to it at leisure more and more.

New to the newly built school, I feel like I do not stick out, but in fact, most students knew other students from their old schools. About a year after the school first opened, we had a ceremony for the person the school is named after. She is here. Am I like her? Her Blackness is highlighted among the sea of White faces that make up the school leaders. Where are the other Black people like her? Mrs. Fiest reminds me of the difference between my old home and this new one. Here there are only two or three other Black kids in my grade and me. I was only in the same room with other Black kids during lunch or PE. The only one I remember clearly is Nick.

After months of seeing White girls with flowing golden or chestnut hair reaching for each other's hair, as a source of amusement and curiosity, these same girls began to play with each other in another way. They began to whisper about this boy or that boy. Although I started to think about boys too, no one ever talked to me about them, except to use me as a conduit to pass a note to another long-haired girl. The paper games that had different names of boys inside, where girls would imagine being paired with this White boy or that White boy. The Asian boys were similarly invisible in these games. Occasionally I was also rendered invisible in this way, although, one lunch, I was moved by a novel aspiration. A nascent desire to have someone to talk with and to whisper to emerged in me. I looked around and saw only one person who I thought I should like. It was Nick, which is a pseudonym like the other names in this chapter, but as soon as the thought of liking him popped into my mind a contrary thought joined it. His freckled face was not pleasant to look at. Were those even freckles or were they moles? The idea formed clearly and slipped away the next moment. Maybe I just wanted to have someone to like. That lunch went by with no one really noticing my unsure declaration, "I think I like Nick," and nothing ever came of it too, except my memories and this story of course.

Being in Girl Scouts led to hanging out with a girl whose parent ran the meetings. Annie was taller than most of us and seemed more mature in other ways. Camping trips meant being finally included in the fun. The more I laughed at Annie's jokes the more she started to let me join her friends for non–Girl Scout get-togethers. Then one day there was a party and a sleepover. Although I had been to their house a few times, this was the first time going beyond the kitchen. Deeper into their home I found a mix of the chaos that I thought characterized my home on a typical day, and there were areas where someone had intentionally straightened up for company. They also had more furniture and home projects than we did. After dinner topped off with cake and ice cream, we talked with her mom about the games we liked most from the last Girl Scout meeting.

As midnight drew near, the talk of going to bed was accompanied with increasing attention to each other's hair again. My hair was the exception of course. No one wanted to braid or brush my hair. And the talk of boys, and who they were starting to like and who they were falling out of liking also seemed to make me invisible. After having gone downstairs to get some water, I lurked on the stairs, not wanting to return to the room and the feeling of exclusion, but unable to go home. I was still friendly with Annie, but I did not continue to go to her house for sleepovers. That was the end of sleepovers for me.

zzzzz

The school bus ride home. I awake and look around. I think the bus has far fewer kids on it than usual. The unfamiliar houses and neighborhood sign confirm my fear. As the bus slows to a stop, I get up to walk to the front. I ask the bus driver where my street is, and they tell me that I missed my stop. It's clear that I have to walk all the way home by myself. The way home is familiar because we are one street away from the entrance to our pine-tree-lined subdivision. Guilt and shame grow and diminishes during the warm walk. I do not know if I volunteered my mistake to my dad when I greeted him.

At home at night, we started making tents and walking on ceilings in our old house in Louisiana, but here, in the two-story house, we perfected it. I would take a large handheld mirror and hold it under my nose to look down onto it. All you can see is ceiling. It made us feel like we were standing on the ceiling and walking around made us feel like we were walking on the ceiling. Approaching a doorway or light fixtures meant we had to step over the visual obstacle and of course the stairs were a real trial. We took turns with usually two mirrors enjoying the subtle sensation of dizziness that came from how this challenged our senses.

To sleep on the floor comfortably, I used the cushions from the upstairs sofa. The TV's VCR held up one part of my tent and the desk held up another part. We took turns being creative in figuring out how to make a tent out of what we had on hand. My sister and I would help the twins, or our parents would oversee their tents. Underneath the makeshift tent is a hybrid territory that partially feels outdoorsy and feels joined with my sisters' tents. Together we are making a novel and adventurous compound of similar structures with familiar sheets and pillows. Safer together, we drift to sleep like much of the lower half of the world slumbers: together on floors. Asleep, or partially asleep, I spot something. It's coming, no, it's right there looking directly at me. A giant suspended spider. Floating inside my tent, it must be maybe three times larger than my head. I jump out of the tent and sprint down the hall where I reach the end just in time for my understanding to crystalize into recognition that nothing was truly there. Was that a dream? A nightmare? Something else? Heart racing, I walk back to investigate the scene, and yes, all is as it should be. Except myself of course, who should be asleep. My sisters are still in their improvised tents asleep, unaware of the foray.

zzzzz

At church. My family started attending different churches occasionally to find one for us to call home. Eventually my little sister announces to my dad that a Black boy in her grade has a dad who is a pastor. When we show up, we sit together and stand when the speaker asks for new visitors. A familiar face catches my eye and we smile in acknowledgment. It's Debra, from middle school. She was always nice to me when I sat near her at lunch although I never got used to the streaks of gray hair that seemed out of place even although something ineffable about Debra always seemed wiser than anyone I knew at this young age. After service, Debra tells me about the youth bible study and how my sister and I should stay for it, to meet and fellowship. It is held next door to the alabaster chapel-like sanctuary. As I walk in, I see two girls who are chatting with one another about the other teens or preteens that seem to be everywhere. Debra introduces us to Jess and Brandy, and Debra explains that we are in the same choir class at school. My sister and I are invited to join the youth church choir, which sings once a month, most months.

That first year, we went to various events with Debra, Jess, and Brandy, and eventually Debra would join us less and less, and then her family eventually joined a different church. Jess and Brandy, though, became good friends that my sister and I looked forward to seeing each Sunday, for choir practice, and during the church summer vacation bible study events. During one of these events, we listened to community leaders who talked about their work and faith. A district prosecutor was introduced to us, and he proceeded to share a message I have heard time and time again in many iterations since. This was the first time it was made explicit to me. He shared how he made it to his position knowing that he needed to be twice as good and working twice as hard as his White counterparts.

Middle school. Some mornings I would wait at home until I heard the afternoon bus screech to a halt at the end of the corner, which was one house away, before leaving, often with breakfast in hand, to catch it. If the weather was cold or raining, this last-minute rush was preferred to uncomfortably waiting outside on the corner or porch. This was why I would occasionally miss the bus and get to school late.

My first class is physical education, so I'm forced to hustle through the empty halls to the girl's locker room to get changed. The rain means we will be doing something new indoors and I am worried I will miss the instructions and be clueless for the entire class period. As I survey the room, searching for a place to sit, I see a girl who seems tall that must be new to the school. She is Black and has a little slouch to her back. I am the only other Black girl in the class. I head to her vicinity somewhat and sit. Turns out she is in seventh grade too, and she has an older sister who is new to the school too. Dee, is what I'll call her here. I had her in another class that day too. I easily find her at lunch, timidly towering over the rest of the seventh graders, and sit with her. She shows me her schedule and I tell her about the other Black students in the grade and school. It turns out that she recently moved into a house that is a few blocks away from ours, and our mutual interest in deciphering the mysteries of Black hair and makeup soon make us good friends.

Among Black friends. Walking home from middle school, after missing the bus in search of Dee's sister, we turned the corner and my focus shifted from the conversation to the houses, to the beautiful weather, and to the meticulous gardens that put our house's standard shrubs to shame.

"Donell keeps acting like he is grown, even though he does not know what he is doing," Dee announces. She often is frustrated at her older brothers who seem to be a part of their house and yet not a part of their house in equal measures.

"I hope he doesn't keep that up," Dee's sister retorts.

"Has he done that before? It seems pretty bold," my sister adds.

"He might have tried to pull that stuff off in our old neighborhood, but Mom is not playing when it comes to this house," Dee adds.

I am listening but not really. I am someplace else but not really.

Eventually someone notices, "Look at Blondie over there in her own world."

I smile, and move closer to their side of the road, to try to join the conversation physically since I do not have anything to add verbally. Last week I told them about how Jess and Brandy gave me that nickname, and how I saw how it was true. I too had also noticed a tendency to be a bit of a space cadet, thanks to an occasional tendency to drift off into my own machinations. Blondes were the butt of jokes those days, and while it was not about being clueless, it was about how I was a little different from my friends and perhaps to them it was an endearing trait. The same way we could, as friends, both comment on and embrace Jess's heroic indecisiveness, or my sister's argumentativeness, this nickname was a way to say they saw my flaws and were okay with them. I could trust them with my flaws because both groups of friends helped break me out of the silent tendencies. These all were traits that could be construed as flaws, but as a group of supportive friends, we were seeing one another as complex individuals. I felt that was never going to happen with the Girl Scout friend, no matter how many sleepovers I went to. In one trip to St. Rose, I visited an aunt's school where many of the students commented about how I sounded White. While it meant little to my prepubescent self, it stayed with me like a subtle crack in a still usable plate of my Blackness. My Black friends and the Black church my family attended affirmed my adolescent identity.

In the early days, before any of us had cars, Dee, her sister, my sister, and I would walk nearly anywhere. One day, we were walking to a fast-food establishment, or a pharmacy, on Highway 6. The absence of a sidewalk did not stop us from walking in the wide grassy strip between the fence and the highway. We were minding our own business, and someone yelled out their car, "N***r." It was clear and loud and directed to us: four Black girls in a largely White neighborhood. I don't think we said much about it. This is likely the first time I am telling the story. Of course, by 2021, the zip code was minority majority, like most of Texas. Race, ethnicity, nationality were rare topics of discussion despite the multicultural educational experiences that shaped so many in this part of the United States in the 1990s until the OJ Simpson chase and the Rodney King video and trial.

MY DIAGNOSIS STORY

At home in 1996. Dad called out, "Dinner is ready" as I entered the house. Instead of going upstairs, I head to the kitchen. I am arriving after everyone else ate already because I had a special choir practice after school. My dad was getting himself a plate too. As I ate, the TV droned on behind us as my sisters watched *Oprah* or some other talk show. As my plate cleared, something changed in me. A heaviness descended on me and soon my senses narrowed. I announce to my dad, who was the only other person at the round kitchen table, "I'm going to pull up this chair and take a nap."

"Christina, don't do that," he pleaded. My dad often calls me by my middle name.

"I can't," I added while pulling up a chair beside me to rest my head on. It was too late.

"You should put your plate up and go upstairs," he persisted, to no effect.

I closed my eyes and was gone, although I could still hear him and the TV drone on unaffected by my departure. I was asleep, but I was also somewhat awake. My senses closed and I was properly asleep for a moment until the rain cleared and the sun dried up all the sleepy wetness that weighed me down moments ago.

As I gradually sat up, my dad said, "You should go take a nap in your room."

Although the sudden urge to sleep was gone, I agreed, and put my dishes away before heading upstairs.

The next day, before I head out the door, my dad tells me about a *60 Minutes* story he saw about narcolepsy. He already talked to my mom about my getting tested, hence later that day my mom made the appointment. About a month later, after two doctor appointments and two sleep tests, it is official: I have narcolepsy. As I learn more about the symptoms, I find they explain the bizarre spider hallucination from years ago. The diagnosis also helps explain why I always seemed to fall asleep during our Sunday morning drives to church or to any place that is beyond our neighborhood. The only time my sleepiness felt *excessive* was the time I fell asleep when we were only a block away from the house. My sleepiness seemed normal at first, but as it subtly grew more frequent and more tenacious, it remained both familiar and unremarkable to both me and my family members. I had begun to sleep away my afterschool hours with little thought about what I might have been missing. Many people who are diagnosed with narcolepsy are fairly oblivious to the sleepiness that has seeped into the cracks and crevices of life.

Now I am put on medication. A small dose of Ritalin. Then it was Adderall, and finally Provigil, which I took for a long stretch of time. Post-diagnosis I was able to stay awake after lunch in math class. Like my mom, I found I was good in math and took four years of classes while in high school. At Spelman, I tested out of math classes and took the GRE several times without ever having taken a college-level math class. My quantitative scores were not spectacular, but they were pretty good considering how long I went without a single math class. I'm jumping ahead again, but thanks to the diagnosis and the search for the right medication to keep me awake, I went from not being able to stay awake in math to being somewhat exceptional at it over the years.

One day my parents told my sisters about the diagnosis and emphasized how, "We just need to make sure Nicole does not do too much driving, and she will be fine."

The next day, I came home after school, and one of my younger sisters was downstairs finishing up a snack. Feeling a little tired, I greeted her and announced that I was going to go upstairs to take a nap.

"Wait," one sister grabbed my hand and pulled me towards the kitchen.

"What?" I asked, hoping she simply needed a hand with reaching something.

"I don't believe it, that you can't control it," she added as if I was hiding something. She seemed to be in denial about my narcolepsy.

She noticed my bookbag and took my notebook from my bag and proceeded to run around the house all while beckoning me to chase her. I tried to keep up with her, but the eleven-year-old was fast and energetic. Dad was downstairs looking at papers or the newspaper, as I caught up to her and claimed my notebook. Nevertheless, she persisted, and now returned to dragging me from room to room, all while sleepiness grew in me despite all the insistent prodding. My narrowing attention went to the velvet-like living room sofa more and more as she dragged me around. It became a tug-of-war between a resistant preteen and a sleepy teen—the sleepy teen won, naturally. Perhaps she could see my energy leaving me as she taunted and pulled on me. My eyes were closed before I was able to curl onto the sofa, finally sliding off my shoes.

"Daddy, tell Nicole to play with me." She was not dissuaded. She merely shifted her strategy.

I was asleep when he replied. It was a short nap, maybe three or five minutes before I had enough energy to go upstairs to my bedroom, which was my initial plan all along. While narcolepsy became a part of my daily life, family communication about it eventually hovered around the topics like driving and medication in my teenage years. I have reason to suspect that the word *narcolepsy* has since fallen from the vocabulary of some family members although they still all seem to understand that I have unique challenges most especially when it comes to doing a lot of driving. While my friends saw it as a possible explanation for my moments of inattention.

zzzzz

Driving, one year later, around one o'clock in the morning.

"Wait a minute, where am I?" I thought, looking at the stop light as my hands gripped the wheel. It was red, and I was stopped, where I should be, but I couldn't remember the whole drive.

Realizing my sister and her boyfriend were in the back of the van lying down, I piped up, "I think I fell asleep."

"What do you mean?" my sister groggily asks.

"I don't remember the drive. I have no idea how I got here."

"Do you need me to drive? Do you need to pull over?"

The light turns green. I turn heading to her boyfriend's house.

"I feel okay, now."

Later adding, "Just know that you shouldn't force me to drive at night ever again."

It was her junior prom, at a school on the other side of Houston, and she wanted to spend the rest of the evening curled up in the back of our turquoise van with her date while I was driving on autopilot. By now I had read about automatic behavior, in Utley's (1995) book, which explained this bizarre symptom of narcolepsy. Although it felt like waking up, automatic behavior means I likely did not go to sleep—rather my brain automatically drove while a part of me, perhaps the parts that create memories, took about a thirty-minute break. It spooked me and my sister. That was the last time she pressured me to drive despite my concerns. Another thing that I learned from Utley is that people with narcolepsy with cataplexy will often suppress their emotions in an attempt to avoid the emotions that tend to trigger cataplexy. This description spoke to me and silently validated the part of me that sought this path. Because as my parents' fights grew louder and more frequent and as my sisters' emotional worlds struggled in this shifting landscape, I found that I was able to pack away my emotions with ease. Amid the year's turmoil that eventually led to my parents' divorce, I often took on the role of the peace-keeper and often thought nothing of myself or of my emotions if it seemed helpful. In rare moments when strong emotions surfaced in me, I learned to turn to my journal to reflect on what was happening and to assuage myself.

SLEEPINESS IN COLLEGE AND BEYOND

Spelman College 1999. This is one of the few classes I am ambivalent about: Introduction to Computers. I enjoyed the majority of my classes, but this one is merely a way to fulfill the science requirement without being in danger of getting a low grade. It is my first semester at Spelman College. While heading back to Abby Hall I'm wondering if my roommate will be there. I am still unsure what happened a few moments earlier. While the professor discussed the reading or something that only partially interested me, something odd happened. Instead of slipping into the sort of embarrassing sleep where you are eventually awoken to the chagrin of everyone in the class, I slipped into a different type of sleep. I slipped partially into sleep, and yet I was still somewhat actively listening. I was waiting for him to ask for questions because moments earlier he reminded me of the question I wrote in the margin of my book. I somehow remained in this enigmatic limbo form of sleep. Not asleep and not awake. In between and bedeviled.

When I arrive to my dorm door, my roommate is there typing away at an essay she needs to submit soon, saying, "I am pulling this out of my ass" which would become her refrain as she solidified her decision to become an English major. Adding, "I wish I could somehow sleep and type this essay. That would be so sweet."

"It's funny you say that, I just fell asleep in class, although I could still hear everything. Once the professor asked for questions, I woke up and offered mine to him," I meekly offered as a curiosity I was still hoping to untangle.

"That is so cool!" she responded, smiling in genuine amazement. She knows about my narcolepsy, but she is turning this into some sort of superpower.

"I hate it," I offered. "I didn't want to be sleepy."

Yet she continued, "So you can sleep through class and still be kind of awake through it. That is the coolest thing I've heard. College would be so easy if I could do that." Invigorated by my superpower, she practically bounces to the downstairs computer lab to print her essay.

After that, I told my professors about my narcolepsy and asked them to be sensitive about how they would address me if I fell asleep in class. To not embarrass me, in short. Thankfully falling asleep in class was rare. There was at least one other time when this hybrid of sleep occurred in which I probably had my eyes open, from straining to stay alert. Part of me slumbered while another part eagerly listened to the lecture and the invitation for questions.

I was fairly scared of falling asleep in public places because of how it rendered me powerless. One day a faculty member forgot about my request and asked me plainly to stay awake during his history class, with the whole class as his witness. I think I felt slightly mortified and somewhat betrayed. I met with him during his office hours soon thereafter to politely remind him of my condition and our conversation at the start of the term. A Black professor with a shiny bald head, he was honestly remorseful about his oversight. I was relieved that it was merely an oversight. At Spelman, constantly surrounded by other brilliant Black people, I never felt like anyone ever stereotyped me because of how I talked. Each classroom and dorm hallway had both women who were raised in Black neighborhoods and women raised in White neighborhoods; sprinkled among us were a few international students who helped us expand our understandings of Blackness and allyship. Here I was simply a narcoleptic, who wrestled with the condition in a space where others saw my humanity and did not confuse sleepiness for anything else than that.

Spelman College fall 2000. History of Social Thought class. I am sitting in a wooden desk trying to tuck my feet under my legs, like I did when I was in high school. It was a way to warm my frigid feet. Black females, who are most of the class, trickle in while the lone Morehouse student sat in his usual spot in the back. As the room starts to seem full, the professor starts to go over what we should be thinking about for our next papers. I have my notebook out and the book beside me. During his preliminary remarks I start to finish a doodle I started in the last class. He is Dr. Weiss, and yes, like his name, which means white in German and Yiddish, he is one of the White male professors at an all-female Black college, but his short stature and gentle yet upbeat demeanor are what really make him stand out from all the professors I've had thus far.

As he turns to write something on the board, he tells us, "Let me apologize in advance if I spell something wrong. I usually avoid writing on the board because I have dyslexia."

My doodling pauses as I take in what he is sharing with us. He goes on to tell us how this simply means he learned to work harder before returning to talking about social theory. During and after the class my mind returned again and again to what he shared. I also think about my family and the dyslexia and other learning challenges many of them overcame or are constantly overcoming. Only now can I put Dr. Weiss's candid admission beside the more silent expressions of living with learning disabilities I became accustomed to through my family members. The Black people in my life, who have dyslexia or other learning conditions like Dr. Weiss, also have worked extra hard to overcome their disadvantages, although they more often will do so silently because being part of what Wilkerson (2020) calls the subordinate class means that deficiencies like learning disorders were less opportunities for empathy, than they were ways to justify cruelty, exclusion, or derision. While at Spelman, I often chose to share my condition with friends, faculty, and sometimes acquaintances. The Atlanta University Center meant being constantly surrounded by people who respected and appreciated Blackness, in all its forms, so I seldom felt I needed to hide who I was. But it was not all sunshine and rainbows in Atlanta. When a neighbor claimed that narcolepsy was imaginary his words wounded me and I oscillated between tending these wounds and feeling frustrated. His frigid conviction that somehow narcolepsy was "in my head" was a shadow that hovered over each subsequent moment when I considered sharing my condition with someone.

University of Tennessee at Knoxville (UTK), summer 2002. I feel it creeping in; I sit up straighter. I put my feet on the floor and sit up from the back of the chair to make myself uncomfortable to keep the whisper of sleepiness away. It is the final day of presentations and thankfully I made it through the summer without any weird moments where I fell asleep unexpectedly. I practiced my presentation and am going after the next person. I feel stress and pressure pulling at me.

Standing in front of the lecture hall, looking at the faces of students and faculty, I pause. Oh no! This is not happening; but it is happening. My mouth opens and everyone knows what this is. The director of the McNair Summer research program at UTK looks constipated as he begins to register the gesture. I swallow the temptation to apologize and start my presentation on the films I analyzed with the American Studies professor that summer. This yawn, and the director's look of disappointment, lodge in me. He knows about my narcolepsy, but this does not stop him from judging me and my yawn.

zzzzz

Summer 2005. London. I am visiting my sister who is studying abroad. Each time I tell fellow American tourists that I am a graduate student who studies the social dimensions of sleep they respond with questions and fascination. Eventually, I begin to sense an opportunity to dialogue about my life with narcolepsy. Nonetheless, each time I decline the implicit or explicit invitation, choosing instead to talk about historical aspects of sleep and culture. These nondisclosures participate in a silent dialogue about sleep and narcolepsy that I am beginning to grow tired of. This silent dialogue cross-examines the mixed feelings I have about the risks and benefits of speaking about my narcolepsy. I conclude that if ever I am going to experiment with talking openly about narcolepsy, strangers who I may never see again are perfectly suitable interlocutors.

On my flight back to the states, I am given the rare luxury of flying across the Atlantic Ocean on standby in a first-class seat. The charming portly White American that sits beside me is more than willing to introduce me to all the perks of my unexpected upgrade—the warm towels to wash my hands, the gourmet menu, the endless free mini bar, and the many snacks available on call. Thousands of feet in the sky I take a risk that I had rarely taken before. In exchange for opening up about his trip and his life, I tell my graying seatmate about my thesis research and finally when he asks what brought me to that line of inquiry—I share the truth about how my life with narcolepsy led to me asking questions about societies' attitudes about sleep. At this stage in my life, I only had one negative experience with disclosing my condition with new acquaintances, yet that was enough to make me averse to discussing narcolepsy with strangers. Yet, in this suspended metal tube surrounded by the privilege and comfort that luck awarded me, I am finally willing to share this part of me with someone I met a moment ago. I think his reaction was a mixture of curiosity and politeness. Over ten years later, as I dust off this excavated memory and place it beside what sleep means in airplanes, I discover how planes are places where the unpredictable sleep of narcolepsy fits—it is a place where, if only for a few minutes, rows and rows of awake and alert people find themselves seduced by circumstance to move between states of sleep and wakefulness in unpredictable and predictable ways. This is a place where narcolepsy blends in with all the other bodies.

Over the course of my late twenties and thirties, my experience of excessive daytime sleepiness, memory problems, and disrupted sleep gradually worsened, and I was largely unaware of this change as were the doctors I saw. I offer this part of my story as an example of the types of absences narcolepsy creates in the lives of those it touches. Once again, sleepiness chipped away at my days without raising an alarm—this is how it works in the lives of many people. This project provides some of the missing pieces by pausing life to tune into the everyday and analyze what might otherwise go unremarked. By revisiting seemingly innocuous sites where my sleep and communication about narcolepsy occur, my narratives suggest that place circumscribes what bodies can and cannot do through the social relations that bring a place into existence.

zzzzz

The second time I was fired for being too sleepy should not have come as a shocker. I should have learned by now, that the catch-22 of being narcoleptic and needing health insurance as a Black woman in the South was going to be difficult. Texas is an at-will state meaning employers can let go of employees for nearly any reason. Someone with narcolepsy does not have to actually fall asleep at work to be fired. I found myself nodding off instead of going over the script for the dating service we were selling that week. I had yet to connect on a personal level with anyone in the office, but I could not ignore what was happening. I felt forced to ask for a moment to myself. We are allowed one bathroom break in addition to a lunch break if we work an eight-hour shift. If it is not a full shift, we could go to the bathroom once.

I paused my calling system and went to the assistant manager who was in the conference room with the door ajar. I did not know what I was going to say until I opened my mouth. "Hey, I have this condition that means I can get sleepy all of a sudden. I felt it coming on and wanted to see if I could just take a five-minute break." Adding, "It's called narcolepsy."

Still sitting, she replies, "I see, um. Can you give me a second?"

I walk back to my cubicle, but I don't want to sit. It might lead to sleep.

"Can you take a seat and I will be right there," she says, looking at the others more than myself.

I sit. Straightening my back to keep sleepiness at bay.

Now the worry starts to eat at me. I could have simply used the bathroom break, but what if I really needed to go later? Did I ruin my chances here? The golden-haired assistant manager called our office manager because this was her first week since being promoted from being on the phones like the rest of us. She had no idea what to do with my question. Time began to crawl as my mind started to race. Sitting at my computer, I can only look into the office as they talked on the phone. I did not feel good about this.

"Okay" it sounded like she said as she opened the door and walked up to my minicubicle. With her usual casual demeanor she said, "Just take the rest of the day off."

This could not be a good reaction to asking for a short break. I also protested because I needed the hours. It felt like this was some sort of punishment although her calm nonchalant attitude made me unsure.

All she could say was, "Just get some rest and come back tomorrow ready to work."

Maybe I should have mentioned my narcolepsy earlier before getting sleepy. It was clearly too late to do anything now. The damage was done. The next day, still feeling unwanted by my employers, I was running late for what might have been the second time since being hired. I called to let them know that I might be five or ten minutes late and that is when the office manager told me to not bother coming in. They had their three strikes against me they needed to justify firing me. I was both stolid and somewhat devastated, again. I loathed the work I had done and was ambivalent about the people there but being fired like that was humiliating. If I could not keep a job that was as basic as telemarketing, how can I expect to get and keep a job I will enjoy, not to mention one that will provide health insurance?

At this point in time, for the last few years, I had been getting my medication from a patient assistance program. My neurologist who needed to sign off on my application saw my tax return and decided to only charge me a $75 copay once or twice a year. Later I would learn that since the doctor and his staff were Muslim, he likely said that I would be Sadaqah, which means charity and is one of the five pillars of Islam. Although I had a master's degree, I went from job to job, to a temp agency, to unemployment, to substituting and to dabbling in self-employment as an Amazon bookseller, before returning to a job that kept me motivated and kept me on my feet—which kept sleepiness at bay. I was standing next to a glowing wall-size photograph of an awe-inspiring autumn shot of a Japanese Maple tree in the Peter Lik photography gallery, in the Houston Galleria, when I checked my email and saw the email from Ohio University. My knees went weak when I read the words of acceptance and congratulations. I was accepted into the PhD program and had funding through a teaching assistantship. This opportunity could be an end to the charade of pretending that I could manage keeping a job long enough to earn health insurance. And yet, it was the beginning of the charade of hoping to selectively hide my narcolepsy in my everyday life while attempting to write about it.

zzzzz

Spring 2015, Ohio University PhD seminar. Is it Jim's seminar or maybe it was Bob's class on quantitative research methods? We are each doing simple micropresentations or maybe it was a class discussion? Either way, I am standing in front of the room of graduate students—my cohort plus maybe one or two other grad students—and of course the professor. Grabbing a marker and readying to write the word I said moments ago onto the board, I stop as the word slips away. The four or five letters completely disappear and I am standing there, a PhD student with no known learning disability unable to spell a word like brain, sleep, shame, write, study, or stop. Whatever the actual word was, it is as gone now as it was then, scrubbed from my memory still. Somehow, I finish what I am saying and head to my seat.

I look towards my roommate in shock as I slide into my chair. She knows that I had maybe four hours of sleep, and about my narcolepsy. I whisper something of an explanation before reengaging with the class discussion. She may have borne witness to my attempts to fight off sleep the night before and may be the only one who might not be shocked by my sudden bout of brain fog. I, on the other hand, was completely caught off guard. I have known about sleepiness getting in the way of learning, but I do not feel sleepy. When I sacrificed sleep the night before, I did not suspect it could impact me in this way. Moving forward, instead of courting sleep deprivation, as a graduate student I began to balance a need for sleep with a habit of testing my limits and adjusting to what I had learned. Going on just four hours of sleep was clearly asking for trouble. I also learned that I could experience brain fog that resembles moments of aphasia in front of a professor and my graduate student peers. This experience caused me to stop to reflect on something I had grown adept at largely ignoring. After all, up until that day, there had been signs, or warnings that something was perhaps amiss, something was malfunctioning, something was changing. Was this the first time during graduate school that I found myself in the middle of speaking while my words slipped from my grasp? If I am being honest with myself, it happened time and time again, in a split second. I usually would try to maintain my face and keep from telling others that my main point disappeared as I was saying it. Being unsure about what exactly was happening meant I could neithereasily save face nor admit what was happening. Was I forgetting my own thoughts right in front of overly judgmental graduate students? Or was I beating myself up? Perhaps both pressures kept me from addressing these minor foibles personally or medically. This time around, I was the person in denial.Telling myself, "Just keep going."

I was in a room of people who were the adult equivalents of Annie and her friends. Their ambivalence towards me and other minorities was now familiar and easily accepted as the norm. I had to hold it together and continue to act like nothing was wrong from day to day and moment to moment. I also hid this pattern from myself as much as I tried to hide it from others. There was no way to know if my brain would take flight daily, weekly, monthly, or just once a semester. The uncertainty inherent in even one of these moments of brain fog was sowing deep-seeded doubts in myself as a scholar. I suspect that these moments are a product of displaced processes that usually occur during sleep. Perhaps the same mechanism that wipes away dreams wipes away active thoughts for people with narcolepsy. This vignette supports the assertion that the social and physical location where narcoleptic symptoms unfold determines how individuals are impacted by these experiences and the overall emotional import they hold in their lives. Being one of two African Americans in my PhD program meant that I needed to get comfortable with White peers fast, even if they never felt comfortable with me. The message drilled into me long ago that I had to work harder than my White peers compounded the pressure I put on myself to stay singularly focused on the goal of finishing my degree program and not to let anything get in the way.

To compensate and to cope with what was happening, I took to writing my reactions and thoughts down during seminars, by hand mostly, using colored pens. I was already taking copious notes, but as I matriculated, notes became an invisible crutch to address the inevitability of brain fog. Should my ideas attempt to jump out of the nearest window as I was speaking, there would be no need to admit it to a room of hypercritical peers; I could glance at my lighthouse to navigate the foggy situation going on in my brain.

zzzzz

Summer 2015. I pull up to a pump and realize that I should move. My gas tank is half full, so I should avoid blocking the pump someone may want to use. I search the gas station for a place to park to finally give into the damp pressure of sleepiness that pulled my eyes down a moment ago. On the side of the store there is a sense of isolation, so I pull beside another vehicle there. Noticing that the truck is empty, I then pull out my sunglasses and my cell phone. It's about 5:30 p.m. How much time do I want this time? How much time do I need? I already had two naps today in the bathroom, which is why I did not expect that sleepiness would still haunt me on my drive home. I set the timer for five minutes, slide on my sunglasses, and relax into the sleepiness that has been subtly numbing my every action.

As the alarm wakens me, I stretch myself somewhat by lifting my head and sitting up straighter. I survey my surroundings. The car beside me is still empty. The sleepy dampness has evaporated. I feel alert enough to travel the winding wooded roads safely once again. I keep my naps a secret because my previous experiences have taught me that discussing narcolepsy and naps with an employer can have dramatic consequences. I treasure the fact that in this summer job I get to pass as able-bodied, although I am unable to complete my duties without the help of an occasional five-minute nap. Nevertheless, I avoid driving responsibilities that would put another person in a vehicle with me, which is how I ethically balance my privacy with my responsibility to be safe. My experiences thus far told me not to trust my employers and coworkers with knowing about my condition and its implications.

THE BATTLE AND THE TRUCE

My bedroom January 2017. This morning I awoke to a familiar tingling felt throughout my body. I have come to think of this as the pleasant sensation sleep uses to seduce people into slumber. For me, when night-time sleep lifts, it often leaves little pieces of sleep behind—parts of sleep that narcolepsy unbinds. I smile widely, enjoying the fleeting moment of happiness and pleasure, and then I hear my cat give a questioning meow, "Are you up?" This is before the more persistent meows that seem to say, "Now! Now! Feed me now!" She sits and waits to see what will happen. Opening my eyes to see my white semifluffy cat, with one blue eye and one amber eye, I meekly exclaim to her, "You are so adorable!" Not placated, she stares back.

Perhaps she can hear me breathe—that must be how she could sense my awakening. Her confidence slowly builds as she starts to inch farther into my bedroom. A few years ago, I forbade her from being in here when I am asleep because her licking and scratching can easily wake me. Nevertheless, she is still allowed to be my immutably reliable alarm clock. My phone informs me that in two minutes the alarm will sound. Rather than feeling grateful or surprised, it is as though those two minutes of sleep were stolen. Turning towards the day, my mind begins to contemplate writing. Brisk air captures my attention as my alarm goes off. Once I sit up, my cat bursts out the door towards her bowl, only to return for her slow fumbling human.

These days, I generally move slowly upon rising out of bed. To evade the sleepiness that might seek to tackle me if I lingered even a minute too long in bed, I used to physically jump out of bed upon waking. Alas, my low blood pressure makes me black out or get dizzy when I attempt such stunts. After I sit up, I linger until my cat's meow coaxes me completely out of bed.

"Yes, I am coming," I say as she paces in front of her bowl continuing her song.

After feeding her, I pick out a pair of pants and a long-sleeved shirt to go for a run. Looking at my bed, I pause, recognizing that if I sit on my bed I might lay down and fall asleep soon thereafter. The risk turns out to be manageable, and now that my chilly feet have socks, the warm bed loses its allure. I turn to my cell phone again. It is remarkable how my cell phone pulls on me. How the room also pulls me. I pick up the sleep log and note yesterday's eating times and how long I slept. I put an "M" for meal in the present hour. I am trying to talk myself into sticking with the plan of getting up to write and eat before going for a run. Then I also put an "E" for exercise two hours later in hopes that I will be ready for a three-mile run by then.

The smell of oatmeal and green tea accompany me as I take a seat in front of my laptop. While eating, I review what I sketched out the night before. Noticing the email application is open, I close it to avoid the potential distraction. Soon I am compelled to Google something, and that thought is accompanied with a desire to also check something else online—these impulses remind me to turn off my Wi-Fi to help me focus on writing. This usually works. No internet means such impulses are restrained. However, this time something else is getting in the way of writing. Where are my words? Then my eyes become heavy and close. I open them and I realize I am too sleepy. But I just woke up! I don't want to go back to my bed. I had seven hours of sleep and a lot of reasons to not be sleepy, but they mean nothing when you cannot think. Cues to act, write, and do are not getting processed; there is nothing "there" where my words should bubble up. It takes a moment to recognize what is happening—the fog of sleepiness has rolled in and now I am stuck, surrounded by an impenetrable muted grayness. I am unable to move.

I exhale, deciding to return to my bedroom, and feeling defeated. And yet I recognize this is the luxury of the weekend. Who decides to wake up at 5:30 a.m. on Saturday? Yet I know that this pull to get back in bed is not a luxury, it is narcolepsy. It also is perhaps yesterday's choice to lie in bed until 9:00 a.m. coming back because the choice to stay in bed yesterday created a pattern that my body thinks it should follow today. Sleep hygiene includes maintaining behaviors that help tell the body when to sleep and when to be awake. Many people with narcolepsy, like myself, will spend a lot of time and energy trying to maintain good sleep hygiene, even if it means waking up at 5:30 a.m. on the days I do not teach at 7:30 a.m. When you have a body that does not naturally separate sleep and wakefulness, this part of the day can at times be difficult.

My run will have to wait. I lie down without changing clothes and let sleep in. I awaken over an hour later to a cacophony of ideas about how good the run will feel and the things I should do today. To me, these are also pieces of leftover sleep. They come with a sprinkle of inertia mixed with diluted inattention that compels me to be still and pay attention to the thoughts that are forming and drifting through me, taking shape and dissolving into one another. This is also the part of narcolepsy that is a gift, one of its gifts—upon waking sometimes my brain is still in overdrive. During sleep the brain reaches levels of activity that exceed what it is capable of while awake; the porous boundaries between sleep and wakefulness mean that I often am able to use naps to access what I call my committee of sleep. If I have a dilemma I must sort out, I might try to take a nap or wait until the morning to see what my committee of sleep comes up with (Barrett, 2001). While I do not always need a nap to access this heightened state of mental activity, it is not something I can easily create, much less control.

My inert body briefly moves into and out of sleep without preamble or warning—especially when this body is in bed. If I am lying down, not only am I in danger of falling asleep, but when this happens the only thing I am aware of is awaking. The memory of falling asleep, as for most people, is a memory that gets erased. The urgent thoughts that invigorate me while keeping me in bed are tucked away although they are in danger of being erased. At the onset of the sleep cycle's process of memory consolidation, the moments preceding sleep may disappear (Dement, 1999). Perhaps if people could recall the experience of *falling* asleep—the gradual loss of perception, thinking, feeling, and action—sleep would seem less appealing. Often my experience of sleep is a type of absence that can be deeply felt.

As I sit in bed again, I think about writing this section of this chapter and realize this room, this story, this bedroom, is an example of what I am hoping to communicate. The choice to paint the walls a muted yet bright yellow was in recognition of the mutual interdependency I have with this space. Its walls influence me and I influence the walls. It changes me and I change it. The place where I might decide, more often than not, to don clothes that overcompensate for my nonmale non-White neurodiverse body is also a scene where I communicate about narcolepsy. It is a place where I can interrogate ableist lies about laziness and also call on them to get me out of bed. This is a place where my submission to sleepiness matches hegemonic expectations about where sleep and sleepiness belong, even though it means something entirely different to me at this moment.

My narcolepsy conspires with the room to allow certain understandings of narcolepsy. Hence, my daydreaming and roaming thoughts—no matter how seemingly fruitful, urgent, or insightful they may be—are also a Trojan horse. Yet, sometimes my self-talk is more pragmatic. Knowing that staying in bed after waking up is correlated with depression means that I avoid this because narcolepsy's number one comorbidity is depression (Zamarian et al., 2014). Over time, I have learned that getting up early with a sense of purpose helps avoid lingering and the naps that accompany it. While in my room and in my bed, sitting still has come to mean that I might be inviting sleep back into my morning. And this is how the active agent—my alert and aware self—starts to disappear. Is *sitting* on my bed tolerable? How can I know that I will not get sleepy while doing something else? Only in this room is it completely socially acceptable to openly recognize the way that narcolepsy is a force with a great deal of agency and control in my life. In my bedroom it is tolerable to strike deals with narcolepsy and to sometimes come out short. These intrapersonal dialogues are acceptable because sleep and sleepiness belong in bedrooms. It is fine when it is a weekend and I do not have to be somewhere soon. It is even okay if the day begins with this type of defeat—trading in my plans for an unexpected nap.

Here in the bedroom self-talk about choices and excuses can fail or succeed. Ableist thoughts surface as negative self-talk, and it succeeds when it creates stress and guilt around sleepiness or sleep. Resentment, shame, and negative thoughts about narcolepsy are more or less muted in my bedroom when I succumb to sleep where ableist Western social norms says it belongs. Ableist negative self-talk fails when we—narcolepsy and me—have a truce and I am able to start the day without a sense of disappointment in being unable to execute the elementary task of waking up. In this way this room allows me to start the day before my feet touch the floor. My understanding of narcolepsy and my sleepiness are mediated by the purpose and intimacy of the bedroom.

Many of the above ruminations were quickly jotted down as I sat in my bed under my teal down-filled duvet. These types of ruminations belong here—on this page, in this sanctioned place of repose. Such negotiations and truces mark neurological differences when they occur in other places—at work, in the car, or in class. These places require an answerability that does not always recognize the way that sleep makes uninvited intrusions in my life. Sleep cannot *do* anything in these places. Public places require another way of communicating about what *people* can and cannot do. In other words, the private and fraught negotiations about whether I should or should not nap in my car or on bathroom floors are challenges that I cautiously disclose here in these pages because initially the comfort and peace of my bedroom granted me a rare bravery. The space imbued me with a courage I too often lack. Moreover, this powerful elixir reaches me at a time when I could not begin to discuss such decisions with the people in my life or with the people I work with.

Spring 2017. Intercultural communication. Students are answering questions about Nick Walker's (2013) essay, "Throw Away the Master's Tools:

Liberating Ourselves from the Pathology Paradigm." The pathology paradigm implies there is a "right" or "healthy" human brain, and if your brain functions in a way that diverges from the dominant "normal" brain, there is something wrong with you (Walker, 2013, para. 12). Like the social model of disability, as an autistic person, Walker urges people to reject oppressive and limiting ways of thinking about one's own brain.

After talking about the earlier concepts in the reading, I introduce the students to the word *neurodivergent* and explain that "This is the word that I like to use when I talk about how my brain is different." I then transition into discussing narcolepsy, all while avoiding my story in particular because I am still too anxious to discuss my story with my students, and because I am worried about end of term evaluations. At this point in time, I am cautious like my dyslexic sister, although I want to be brave like Dr. Weiss. Then, after talking about narcolepsy briefly, I share the viral video *What Narcolepsy Really Looks Like. Spoiler Alert—It Sucks* (Sleepy Sarah Elizabeth, 2014). This video features a White red-haired, college-aged woman who experiences several falls and near falls as a result of narcolepsy with cataplexy and sleepiness, all creatively captioned to indicate what was happening from her perspective. The video quickly circled the globe in 2014 and was highlighted on TV news as a rare authentic glimpse into an often-misrepresented condition. I am using this video of a White woman, because it is interesting, and because I am unconsciously aware of the way that even hints of Black disability are potent enough to evoke stereotypes of laziness, Welfare Queens, social security truancy, etc. I want to share more, but I am still too scared of negative feedback on evaluations, suspicious whispers, and awkward jokes to be more vulnerable today.

We were able to start the next day with a question-and-answer session about narcolepsy. Embracing my hidden disability in this albeit somewhat defensive and indirect way nevertheless invited discussions and papers in which students spoke candidly and critically about their own neurodiversity—anxiety disorder, ADD, and ADHD. One student used her final essay to write about how she used to think that there was something wrong with her, but now she is working on accepting herself and her anxiety disorder in a way that recognizes the harm in internalizing ableist ideas. As an instructor, I felt grateful and fulfilled that I was able to help a student turn off the negative self-talk that many people with hidden disabilities live with. The process of learning about disability and modeling a healthy relationship to one's body and pathologies is never-ending. Despite my reticence about discussing my narcolepsy, I can perhaps still teach in a way that transforms the classroom into a space where bodies are not compulsively measured and compared.

zzzzz

Narcolepsy unfolds in lives that are impacted year after year by the way others respond to their particular embodiment. Men with narcolepsy, White, Black, or of another race or ethnicity, will have a different story that is impacted by how they were taught to deal with vulnerability. Other Black women with narcolepsy will have different racial identities and different attitudes towards talking about the condition. During my PhD program, and for as long as I can recall prior to then, I was very much under the influence of what is called Black Super Woman syndrome. This is where Black women are afraid of sharing weaknesses and vulnerabilities and as a result miss out on opportunities for connection and support (Woods-Giscombe et al., 2019; Woods-Giscombé, 2010). The evolution of my identity as a Black woman is connected to the places where I found myself. As I approached the support group which included mostly Black and White participants, I evaluated my approach to race in the questions I asked and decided to take a fairly colorblind approach to the topic. This reflected my approach to other research I conducted and the general pre–George Floyd attitude towards race in much of the communication research I used to guide my work. This autoethnography reflects a post–George Floyd era of institutions and individuals with an increased willingness to wrestle with issues of race and racism in both personal and systemic contexts. Since finishing my PhD, I changed from a woman who was dreadfully afraid of sharing my everyday experiences with narcolepsy into one who mostly has situational reservations. I also have since received better medicine that better controlled the numerous bouts of EDS contained in this chapter. The next chapter focuses on the experiences of someone who was newly diagnosed with narcolepsy while also exploring what it means to have narcolepsy while at work more generally.

Chapter 3

At Work with Narcolepsy

People with disabilities face overt and indirect forms of employment discrimination because of reservations some may have about their capabilities (Scheiber, 2015). An example of one negative attitude towards people with narcolepsy appeared in a story about Nicole Jeray, a professional American golfer who also has narcolepsy. A *Golf Digest* article about her includes a quote from her doctor saying, "people with a severe condition like hers almost always have a difficult time achieving in life. It's no accident that through history, there are almost no famous persons known to have suffered with severe narcolepsy" (Diaz, 2001). He goes on to praise Nicole's personality, attitude, and determination, in a manner that is somewhat oblivious to the possibility that Nicole might disprove his faulty assumptions about the prospects of people with narcolepsy. Both negative attitudes and low expectations are a major barrier people with narcolepsy face inside and outside of work environments. When a doctor feels comfortable sharing his low expectations and having them published widely, it suggests that these ideas may be prevalent in the discourse at large and in the lives of people with narcolepsy.

Contrary to what the doctor quoted above claimed, there are many examples of prominent people throughout history and alive today who can be characterized as being notably prone to irrepressible daytime sleepiness, which is a more historically useful way to describe narcolepsy. The most notable historical day-sleepers would be Thomas Edison (Opie, 2009), Winston Churchill (Brody, 1994; Haltom, 2015), and Harriet Tubman (Crewe, 2007). Thomas Edison turned to naps to help him figure out complex problems (Opie, 2009). Going further back in time there is Dante Alighieri's *Divine Comedy* which includes complaints that resemble the symptoms of narcolepsy, suggesting that he himself had narcolepsy with cataplexy (Plazzi, 2013). Since the term *narcolepsy* was coined in 1879 (Nicholls, 2018), precautions should be taken against hastily comparing those whose symptoms suggested a pathology to those who have been diagnosed and treated.

Well-known people with narcolepsy who are alive today include the host of the late-night show *Jimmy Kimmel Live* (Gross & Kimmel, 2013); George Church, the Harvard geneticist (Guturu et al., 2016; Herper, 2009); Henry Nicholls, renowned science writer and author of three books (Nicholls, 2018); and Harold McEwen Ickes, White House deputy chief of staff for President Bill Clinton (Lewis, 1997). Danielle Brooks, an educator and narcolepsy advocate, created the website www.SucceedingwithNarcolepsy.com to highlight successful people with narcolepsy and to counter limiting messages about it (Brooks, 2013). While in high school, she published her story and the stories of many others who are living successful and fulfilling lives with narcolepsy to counter negative messages she and others encounter (Brooks, 2013). Julie Flygare is perhaps the most visible patient advocate in the United States. Through Flygare's (2013) memoir *Wide Awake and Dreaming,* her blog, her Narcolepsy Not Alone photo campaign, her nonprofit organization Project Sleep (Project Sleep, n.d.), and many opportunities to speak about narcolepsy, Julie's work advocates for a better understanding of narcolepsy while also being the public face of narcolepsy in the United States. She is extraordinarily active which is another powerful testament to what can be accomplished while living with a condition like narcolepsy.

Furthermore, people with narcolepsy are educated at a rate comparable to that of non-narcoleptics and in the United States they marry at comparable rates as well (Black et al., 2014; Cohen & Mudro, 1992; Flores et al., 2016). On the other hand, people with narcolepsy are twice as likely to develop psychiatric conditions, and their utilization of medical services is many times greater than the non-narcoleptic (Black et al., 2014). Yet, such numbers are limited in what they can convey about the impact of living with narcolepsy. In a population-wide study of narcoleptics in Italy, after researchers collected and analyzed their data, they mused that, "It would be interesting to understand why [narcolepsy with cataplexy] had a greater impact on the social lives of patients than on their education and employment" (Ingravallo et al., 2012, p. 1298). To answer this question, and to address the issues that lay at the heart of this study, this chapter presents a rich description of how the experience of narcolepsy at work is tied to the specifics of place, personal history, and social resources.

This chapter presents narratives of the interview process to blend and experiment with both qualitative and ethnographic writing. By sharing the story of the interview, the work of interviewing becomes a sensory experience that has affective potential for readers. Storytelling is a way to place the reader in the room with the two people with narcolepsy who are both struggling to understand our own lives more fully. Using the transcriptions, photographs, sensory fieldnotes, video, and descriptions from audio recordings, the vignettes seek to convey a rich situation where knowledge is discovered through engagement with both the context and story. As a researcher and a peer with narcolepsy, these two roles become two distinct voices in much of the book. The peer is the voice of the interviewer who sought to create conversations within the context of an interview. The researcher, however, is the voice of the person who transcribed the interviews, creating a fabricated form of intimacy that only transcribers may understand. It also reflects the insights gained from analyzing the transcripts for themes.

Embedding meanings within a rich and embodied exchange yields accounts of narcolepsy that are always and at once bound to the specific nuances of the chimerical moment. The narrative form invites readers to discover what I and my conversational partner discovered about each other and narcolepsy by providing some of my analysis in the story. The story of the interview is followed by a discussion of the themes and how they shed light on what was gleaned. The discussions also revisit other interviews to shed light on the relationship between narcolepsy, work, and place.

zzzzz

When I rushed into Strongwater, about ten minutes late, I smiled widely because I saw that this was not going to be like last month when no one showed up—several people were here already. I met Penny, Elaine, Cameron, John, Jane, and Cynthia that morning. Early in the meeting we learned that Penny, a twenty-nine-year-old White woman, is new to narcolepsy—having been diagnosed at the beginning of the year. During our meal, Penny introduced her husband to the group by saying, "He doesn't think it is 'real,'" in a cadence and tone that was upbeat. No one said anything in response as she continued to explain how he just thinks she is "lazy." I did not detect any sour overtones that might have indicated sarcasm—I was hoping it was a joke which is why I scrutinized her face for a cue to laugh. Perhaps it was supposed to be a joke between Penny and her husband that she was letting us in on. I checked to see how others reacted and they acted like nothing happened. I was confused. Initially I suspected she was being passive aggressive, which further confounded me. Yet Penny was describing an experience that I was all too familiar with; however, her attitude and frankness was jarring because I had become used to hearing people wrestle with issues of legitimacy with clear feelings of despair and discontent.

Unfamiliar with Columbus, I was unsure which part of the city the GPS navigated me to, but I was able to find Penny's house without too much trouble. The stucco house is golden clay-colored with two off-white garage doors and a driveway that can fit about half a dozen or more vehicles. The backyard spills out from the driveway without any clear beginnings or endings between the parts of their property space and the property it buttresses.

After I pulled up, I got out my pad folio and the folder that had one of every sheet I needed. I then made sure I had a writing utensil and, after turning off the GPS function instead of putting my phone away, I realized that I could take a photo of something to better recall the details of the day—I forgot to take photos before and after my first interview. This was a second chance. I shyly took a picture of the garage and what might be her backyard and worried that someone might be able to see me although no one was in sight.

At the window-less front door, I rang the doorbell and started to wonder about what my plan was if no one answered. Thankfully that question was abandoned as soon as it was taken up when I was enthusiastically greeted by Penny as she reached for her oversized puppy, Adam. He is a golden brown Leonberger puppy and looks like he weighs around one hundred pounds. He has not yet learned how to jump and just yesterday learned how to stand on his hind legs to try to get to a higher space. He reminded me of a teddy bear but with floppy ears and fluffy tan fur that darkens to black around the face and paws. Unlike most puppies I've met, this one does not bark and does not force himself into my space. He seems only mildly curious.

This chapter will focus on my time with Penny, who wanted to do her second interview at work to talk about her struggles of having narcolepsy while at work. A newly diagnosed woman with narcolepsy with cataplexy, Penny's diagnosis story came after previous diagnoses of ADHD, anxiety, and depression. Penny's doctors saw her accounts of falling asleep on stimulants as a sign she may have a sleeping disorder. She is a speech pathologist at an elementary school and spent the fall semester of the current school year undiagnosed with narcolepsy symptoms. Since it can take months or even years to determine the right medications and dosages to help control the symptoms, Penny still experienced moments of excessive daytime sleepiness, memory problems, concentration problems, and had a mild cataplectic attack after beginning treatment. Penny's story highlights three dimensions of experiencing narcolepsy at work: (1) the presence of onlookers should one become sleepy or take a nap; (2) the difficulty of working with sleepiness, inattention, and other impairments; and (3) the inflexible and flexible dimensions of work and its environment. Penny talked about several strategies she has for dealing with sleepiness. Although work was exhausting and inflexible, Penny was enthusiastic in her attempts at educating those she worked with about narcolepsy and had the support of close colleagues that let her nap in their classrooms. This chapter also integrates accounts of working with narcolepsy as discussed with the other participants to show a range of perspectives and experiences.

PENNY'S DIAGNOSIS STORY

Penny walked me to the circular wood-laminate table, which I can see was washed with a wet rag a moment ago. The table still looked wet, which is why I was reticent about sitting down. I needed a dry spot for my computer, or maybe I should only use my smartphone. Rather than bring this up, I decided to use my phone to record the interview as I took my seat.

During the interview, I learned that her earlier claim from yesterday's support group meeting—that her husband "thinks I am lazy"—was not a joke. Still, she maintained an upbeat manner in general and seems to find it funny that the people closest reject her narcolepsy. It seemed she was at home alone; halfway through the interview she mentions that her husband was in the other room. During the interview, Penny got up a few times to tend to the puppy who liked to put his paws in his drinking water. When that became tiresome, he dumped it out and contentedly laid in the water.

My first question for Penny and all my interviewees was, "What is your diagnosis story?" Penny's diagnosis story starts with being treated for ADHD, as discussed previously. Penny thought "this ADHD stuff" has been there since she was a toddler. Penny also had memory issues as a kid. She suspected that her discussions of her memory issues are what pointed her psychologist to ADHD. She explained, "I can't remember anything. I have never been able to remember, and my mom would yell at me and say you need to make a list. And I'd say I made a list, I forgot to look at the list." She went on to say, "I know everyone at the group said that's all narcolepsy, but the narcolepsy stuff started later," and she also attributed the executive functioning issues she has been dealing with to ADHD, too.

I was fascinated by her story. As I listened to her, I started to suspect that, like many others with narcolepsy, she was misdiagnosed for years but at this point, about six months after the diagnosis, she did not see this prior diagnosis as a misdiagnosis (Kryger et al., 2002). She then told me about how once she was on medicine for ADHD she could, "take data." She explained,

> I couldn't take data, and the session with the kid—I couldn't transition from one thing to the next because they'd all say, "Well you need to be thinking about the next thing while you're doing this, so that your transition is better." I said I can't think about the next thing while I'm doing this; if I'm not 100 percent thinking about this, then I'm not doing it.

In graduate school, she learned that she couldn't transition and had other organizational issues. Yet, once put on ADHD medication, she saw improvements, which is why it seemed to be a correct diagnosis.

I saw an opportunity to help her by sharing what I learned about narcolepsy and mental fog,

> I want to, um at times I'll like share a little bit of my story so that it's more conversational, but growing up I was "ditsy." My nickname was "Blondie." And before I was diagnosed, there wasn't a reason, I was sort of like you know, I just forgot stuff. I just said weird things. Sometimes my brain was someplace else. But that's okay because I had better grades than all my peers and was just, they just knew I was brighter—I just wasn't brighter all the time, right?

At this we both laughed. We were both extremely bright women who excelled in school but had odd and undeniable difficulties from time to time. I went on to explain how narcolepsy is a pathology, and unfortunately the cognitive symptoms are not treated like primary symptoms even though it is a part of excessive daytime sleepiness. What many call "brain fog" gets incredibly little attention and treatment, therefore it is difficult to recognize that those early symptoms may have been early signs of sleepiness (Flygare, 2014; *The Voice of the Patient: Narcolepsy*, 2014; Young, 2013).

Penny added, "But then can you have narcolepsy since from being like a toddler all the way up, but then not the cataplexy until later? I don't know."

I responded by explaining, "It's developmental and so it does progress slowly," indicating that the onset of narcolepsy symptoms is usually gradual instead of being a sudden change in sleep patterns and neurological functioning. I also stated, "It's not unreasonable to think that your experiences have a long history even though they didn't result in you falling asleep, because these kind of things you're describing, that is all a part of narcolepsy." I paused, unsure if I wanted to take this detour. Penny encouraged me to continue, so I explained how narcolepsy symptoms are moments when the brain is engaging in processes that should occur during sleep but instead are happening while we are awake.

After talking about my Post-it metaphor of sleep and narcolepsy she revised her earlier understanding, and said, "So then I almost feel I should change my form, on when did it start: question mark."

To which I said, "Okay, yeah you could do that. Here," while reaching for the form. Penny used the black ballpoint pen to scratch out what she wrote and beside it she put a question mark on the form where it asked when they started to experience symptoms.

"Because, like I don't remember a time when I wasn't tired."

"Okay," I replied.

"Even like in middle school or even elementary school, I don't remember ever not being tired." She continued, "I guess, like the cataplexy, and the actually falling asleep didn't start until . . . "

"More recently?" I offered.

"About twenty-two, twenty-three years old." Penny started to think about her past through the lens of narcolepsy and begins to see it differently, realizing, "Um, although I do know that my mom says when I was like in preschool, like I don't remember it, but if I got hit, like bumped my head she said I would pass out." She realized that these memories of passing out could now be understood with the lens of narcolepsy or may have been cataplexy.

"Huh," I said.

She continued, "And then [I would] wake up and be fine, so she'd have to tell people like when they're babysitting or whatever, like if she turns and she passes out, she's fine, don't take her to the hospital."

To which I said, "Wow!" I added that, in my preliminary research in which I did email interviews with people with narcolepsy, there were people who said they are pretty sure they had narcolepsy as a toddler. I also shared how my family has joked about how I was such an easy baby and toddler, because of all the sleeping I would do, that my parents thought having kids was easy which is part of why they had three more babies in the next three years.

Penny added that she has always had "really vivid dreams," otherwise known as epic dreams. She would remember them clearly—even too clearly because, "sometimes I've spent all day going, 'That dream wasn't real, that wasn't a real thing.' I feel like it gets stored in like this was a real thing that's happened, and it's always been like that." We went on to talk about déjà vu and the extra work of separating fact from fiction when dreams can be as vivid as real life.

The confusion we discuss is referred to as dream delusions, which refers to false beliefs that can persist for days or even weeks; they point to unique memory issues in people with narcolepsy that deserve more research and attention (Wamsley et al., 2014). Dream delusions are different from hypnogogic hallucinations because the former occur during sleep, when something goes amiss and these dreams are remembered as a story with such detail and complexity that they may at times seem real (Mazzetti et al., 2010). The language of symptoms may at times feel incongruent within discussions of dreams, yet prior to a diagnosis, merely six months before our conversation, Penny had few words to describe her falling down or her endless lack of energy prior to her diagnosis. Our conversation demonstrated how others with narcolepsy may play a significant role in developing a story about one's body and condition.

Many come to understand narcolepsy through memories and communication about experiences that only later come to have a name. For Penny, before her diagnosis, her "passing out" and her tiredness were not a part of a larger physiopathology. Many of the conversations with my interviewees caused my interviewee or myself to revisit and revise our understandings of our bodies and our pasts. By narrating the interview, I performatively write about these shifts in understanding. As Kristin Langellier (1999) says, "The focus on performance emphasizes the way telling intervenes between the experience and the story, the pragmatics of putting narrative into practice, and the function for participants" (p. 127). Showing both the story and the experience of the telling reveals how my participants' narratives serve both the pragmatic and functional purpose of making sense of narcolepsy. It is likely more adept to acknowledge that I developed a narrative voice that sought to include the perspectives of both the researcher and the researched. In narrating the exchanges I am deploying narrative as, "both a mode of reasoning and a mode of representation" (Richardson, 1997, p. 28). Through narratives we adjusted our understandings of narcolepsy and via narratives I hope to present these moments to my audience.

Many of the people I interviewed and talked with felt left to make sense of narcolepsy as individuals because of the paucity of information their doctor provided. Support groups and online resources often help compensate for what may not fit into a brief doctor's appointment. Upon diagnosis, many people will look at descriptions of narcolepsy symptoms and begin to understand previously unexplained memories in terms of the narcolepsy symptoms. This process of telling a new story about one's body occurs over time and through embodied or virtual conversations become opportunities to revisit and amend previous understandings of narcolepsy, as Penny does here. While Penny's story indicates that she has always been tired and she had experiences that suggest that she might have had cataplexy as a young girl, there is no way to verify or disconfirm this story. At a later meeting, Penny told me that the question of when it started, or what came first, ultimately did not matter. Neat narratives about narcolepsy as a pathology and as a subject of a research investigation fail to reveal the ways that making sense of sleepiness may become a never-ending endeavor for people with narcolepsy.

The narratives of dialoguing about narcolepsy seek to present a heteroglossia of voices (Bakhtin, 1987): the medical jargon, the ethical doctor, the willing interviewee, the pharmaceutical's promise, the multifaceted person, the embodied interviewer, the cautious writer, the vulnerable researcher, and the nascent relationship. All these voices contribute to shaping how individuals may come to understand themselves and narcolepsy. Many may be present in each narrative conversation about narcolepsy in this book. The meaning of narcolepsy in everyday life lies in Bakhtin's (1987) concept of dialogue and "dialogization" in which a culture becomes aware of competing definitions of the same event (p. 427). The meaning of narcolepsy symptoms shifts and transforms because as voices change the meanings change. In seeking to create an account of the meaning of narcolepsy in the words of those who live with it, this is also an attempt to avoid a monologue focused on the author that reflects a singular perspective. The absence of a monologue or singular perspective does not omit the power dynamics that give authors control over what is said and how participants are portrayed. The potential that Penny's initial position could have been initially correct, and the vulnerability embodied in my suggestion that perhaps I could know her history better than she knows her history are voices in the dialogue that should be heard as much as the other parts of the narrative. Several years after this interview, there is clearer evidence about the high prevalence of people with narcolepsy in ADHD groups and vice versa (Wilenius & Partinen, 2020). Doubt and especially self-doubt play a large role in the lives of people with invisible conditions like narcolepsy.

In Paul E. Pfuetze's (1961) book on Martin Buber and Herbert Mead, he declares that, when one is faced with the mystery and uncertainty of illness and mortality, "Either we believe there is meaning in life, or we are engulfed in the tragedy of human existence" (pp. 285–286). Similarly, many people with narcolepsy are galvanized to make sense of life and illness through stories. Each of the following chapters focused on a location presents the diagnosis story of the participant to provide the context for understanding how they experience narcolepsy in specific spaces. Penny's diagnosis and context for further storytelling reveal that she is working to make sense of narcolepsy with little help from her husband and with years of competing diagnoses.

Penny initially wanted to reflect on her time working as a producer in a theater but arrangements to use a space like that fell through. It is also worth noting that in contrast to her current struggles as a teacher, her time spent working in a theater was so invigorating that there was a notable absence of sleepiness. Penny was open to interviewing at the school she worked at to reflect on her experiences of working with narcolepsy.

AT WORK WITH ONLOOKERS, INATTENTION, AND INFLEXIBILITY

My sleepiness was not under control enough for me to plan to drive to and from Columbus as needed for the interviews. Accordingly, I spent the night in Columbus several times during my research to avoid driving while sleepy. Back home, in Athens, I was in the beginning stages of painting my bedroom a soft yellow color, which was inspired by the cheerful walls of one of the hotel rooms I stayed in during my trips to Columbus. The day I interviewed Penny began in one of these hotel rooms. I was complimented on my outfit as I waited behind a father and daughter for the waffle maker. I was wearing yellow pants and a black-and-white-striped cotton shirt and a black sweater. While waiting for the chance to make a waffle, I took a picture of the fruit water the hotel made that included pineapple, lemon slices, and other slices of citruses. I hoped one day I could make it. After breakfast I checked out and headed to meet Penny.

Once I realized my GPS was not helping me locate the school, I pulled into a driveway to make a U-turn. As the cop in my rearview mirror drove by, I called the number Penny gave me. She described how to find the school, but it still took a while for me to orient myself to her instructions. When I finally drove up to the nearly empty parking lot, she was standing outside. The building looked new—it could have been built in the last five or ten years. As she led me to her office, I saw no one. I later learned that this was the day that teachers used to organize their rooms or get rid of old decorations and graded student projects. Penny's room was right down the hall from the entrance, hence I did not see much of the unique school.

Penny had left her oak door open, but once we entered she closed it. We sat at the trapezoid table she uses to work with students. Once I described how this interview will be different from the first interview, in that it would be up to Penny to decide what she wanted to share, I perched my computer on a short bookshelf that faced Penny and started the video and sound recording. She had worked here for one year, and as previously mentioned, she spent half of this school year as undiagnosed. This was the end of the semester when she had been working with a doctor to figure out the right medications to manage her excessive daytime sleepiness and disrupted nighttime sleep.

In the second interview, I had better rapport with Penny, and at the end I was delighted because we both seemed to personally benefit from the experience. Then I made notes about the interview and transcribed it. Interpretive phenomenological analysis (IPA) was used to review the transcript to identify ideas that emerged during the interview and for the rest of the interviews in the book. The largest and most salient IPA clusters became the themes I will explore in the remainder of this chapter (see appendix for more details on this process). Penny's account highlights three dimensions of being at work with narcolepsy: (1) the presence of onlookers should one become cataplectic, sleepy, or take a nap; (2) the difficulties of working with sleepiness, inattention, and other impairments; and (3) the ways in which work can be inflexible in some respects while being flexible in other respects. Within each of the following sections, after sharing Penny's account of being at work, there is a brief discussion of other participants who shared details about the challenge of dealing with narcolepsy amid their work.

The Optics of Naps and Sleepiness

After pressing "Record," I asked, "Tell me again, how is [narcolepsy] a part of being in this space?"

Penny began by saying, "I just started here in August, so this is the first time I've had a job where I have to go all day, like the 9 to 5, five days a week kind of thing. And so I think that's actually been kinda difficult. This is a big jump, but," gesturing towards the closed door that is next to her desk, "it's a very public spot at my desk, in that there is a lot of traffic back and forth," moving her arm left to right while pointing, "because the way to the cafeteria is out this door." She pointed to the right edge of the door indicating that the cafeteria is down the hall to the right. Her solid oak door has a long narrow four-inch window that sits left of the door knob. The desk with her computer sits beside this door to the right. She continued, "And every student in the school goes by. And the way from the dorms is—this door. So, in the morning they all come through; then they all go through for lunch, and come back from lunch; then the evening, people meet out here. It's very public." She is not able to take a nap in her own classroom—ever since I stepped into the room, I suspected that she was able to use this private space to help manage her sleepiness with naps. It turned out to be the opposite because under no circumstances can she block the window. She disclosed, "I always feel like somebody's watching all the time."

In response, I asked, "When did you start to feel that way? When they showed you the room, did you already know that this was going to be an issue?"

Penny talked me through her realization that onlookers are everywhere, explaining, "No, it wasn't until I was sitting at my desk, and I laid my head down," and she put her head on the table to demonstrate. "And I was like, 'Oh, man.'" Lifting her head up, "'Oh I can't lay my head down, I have to lift my head up.'" Then bobbing her head as if she was wrestling with sleepiness, she added, "'Oh, they're all coming back from lunch now, I have to be awake and doing things.'" Although she can't nap in her office, she has a friend whose room has giant floor pillows. When Penny needs a nap, she goes to her friend's room to sneak in a quick nap when the timing is right.

Relieved that she has this type of resource, I probed, "But you still live with fear; it's usually all it takes?"

She explained, "Yeah; it's the fear of it. Oh my God, they're all gonna think I'm sleeping on the job. Afternoons get really tough." Penny went on to explain how if she came to school late, not only does the teacher and student first on her schedule know, but, "Everybody knows when I'm late; if I get here late. All the kids are like already starting to come in, I'm like, 'Excuse me'; unlocking my door." Indicating how she would have to squeeze past a line of students parked outside her door.

I empathized with her and added, "It's like checking in; like when you get to work, some people—the manager will see you, right? So, there's no way of sneaking in. But for you it's not a manager, it's like, everybody."

"Everybody knows; I'm late. Every day. Except today! I was early. I think like all year I've been late; today there's no students and I'm early. It's like, really?"

For Penny and for many people with narcolepsy waking up in the morning is difficult because spending even a moment in bed can cause them to slip back into deep sleep. When I was in college I wrote on a sheet of paper Nike's slogan, "Just do it," to remind me to hurry to get out of bed when I woke up or else risk losing hours to the quicksand of narcolepsy. This quicksand makes waking up tricky and can cause drowsiness, lethargy, and tiredness—leading some people to hope that five more minutes might remove these rubbish feelings. I told Penny about the sign and how I have a cat that is my trustworthy alarm clock because she will not stop meowing and pawing at me until I get up and feed her in the morning. If I get back in bed after feeding her, it is just a matter of time before she would start to try to rouse me again. When I asked about what happens in the mornings, Penny explained that after turning off the alarm, she immediately falls asleep and her dreams keep going like they never stopped. She has learned to avoid morning commitments since she is likely going to miss them. For Penny, being someone with narcolepsy at work often meant being surrounded by people who may become onlookers and witnesses if she were to suddenly fall asleep or experience cataplexy.

These onlookers may take a more active role. Many people find humor in the cataplexy *response.* In reaction to a question about whether she still experiences cataplexy, Penny explained that most of her cataplexy is under control because of the Zoloft her doctor prescribed before her diagnosis. She added that she still has what she calls a "micro sort of cataplexy." Which she went on to describe, "A student startled me the other day and I dropped—I was eating and I dropped my food and they thought it was hysterical." Penny showed me how slight the cataplectic response was by bringing her hands up and weakening her grasp of an imaginary sandwich and continued, "Then she kept trying to startle me and I had to be like 'no,' like 'you have to stop.' They're like, 'Ha, ha, ha,' like 'oh Rebecca, scare her and she dropped her food, oh my gosh.' I'm like, 'No. No this is not a thing. You are not all going to try to jump out at me now. We're finished.'"

Shocked I declared, "So ridiculous!" Her description suggests that the student did not take her request seriously because they continued attempting to scare her, yet she seemed more annoyed than angry. I noted, "It sounds like you have a good attitude about the whole thing." Alternatively, her reaction to this antagonism might be an example of the emotional restraint people with narcolepsy with cataplexy may develop to ward off the emotions that invite cataplexy. Or it could be remarkable because our different races often have different approaches to perceiving and addressing conflict in interpersonal contexts.

"I kept telling her 'no,' like 'that's it.' She scared me like three times in one day, and I finally had to be like, 'If you do that again you'll get lunch detention . . . You're done.'" She was annoyed that this student didn't understand. Penny added that she is glad that her trigger is being startled because falling down is a relatively acceptable reaction to being surprised. The sight of seeing someone fall, drop something, or lose their balance upon being startled doesn't attract the same type of onlookers that other triggers may bring. On the other hand, this trigger may be contributing to her husband's inability to understand her falls as cataplexy and therefore indicating a pathological condition.

To summarize, Penny's experience of being at work with narcolepsy accompanies a sense of surveillance even when she has more privacy than the teachers who do not have doors or walls. Students and teachers are also able to see her tardiness and when she falls behind her scheduled meetings with students. The narrative form unfolds and as it does Penny's understanding of narcolepsy begins to surface. Mornings at work are precarious because of the way narcolepsy delays transitioning to wakefulness. Penny's chronotype and the schedule of schools who teach young children is a significant misfit, but Penny is optimistic about her ability to do better. Prior to starting this job, as a graduate student, the inconsistent schedule may have made it harder to see the type of clear pattern that emerged when she had to be at the same place at the same time for five days a week. In one of her interviews with me, another participant, Nancy, discussed how she was a speech pathologist when she was diagnosed with narcolepsy, but she was eventually fired from that job, which is how she started to work at libraries. While Nancy spent a lot of time working as a librarian, her diagnosis was the beginning of a number of job changes. As she put it, "Once I retired, then I started doing different kinds of volunteer work, volunteering in school libraries and some other places, too. Some were a much better fit for me, partly because it was a shorter period of time." The challenge for people with narcolepsy, and for others who might identify as being neurodiverse, is finding the right niche where their weaknesses can be balanced with opportunities to build and strengthen their assets and talents (Armstrong, 2010). Whereas Nancy discovered her niche when she retired, Penny is at the beginning of her journey with narcolepsy and is optimistic about her ability to find a niche in speech pathology.

The story of a student discovering her cataplexy trigger and then proceeding to try to startle her again viscerally illustrates Penny's unique form of vulnerability. In addition to the visibility of her room, Penny and many people with cataplexy are familiar with how something unpredictable can bring about a cataplexic fall. While Penny was able to eventually put an end to attempts to startle her, the story is a glimpse into how even the most mundane days and places can swiftly transform into a situation that makes it difficult for someone like Penny. The ongoing visibility of sleepiness and cataplexy means that for Penny, at work, hiding this aspect of her body may be an unrelenting effort.

The Flexibility and Inflexibility of Space and Time

Despite the inflexibility of the schedule, there are ways that Penny's needs and the expectations of the job are in alignment. Early in the interview I asked, "Has anybody seen you trying to take a nap, or that moment when you put your head down, did somebody react?"

"No. If I'm taking a nap, I go to my friend's room down the hall, because she has big pillows. So after school sometimes I'll go down and take a nap in her room."

"That's . . . " I struggle to find the right word, "awesome."

Penny added, "I need pillows for here. But no, nobody's ever said anything, so that's good." Sometimes she doesn't need a nap, but instead can simply close her eyes for a few moments, and after that she feels better. Later she described in detail all of the changes to the room she has made since she started at the beginning of the year. Most of the changes reflect an effort to declutter the room and minimize distractions.

I asked, "Does it feel different when you are here with somebody versus here by yourself?"

Penny nodded her head indicating yes while yawning widely before saying, "Yes it does. I tend to stay later than a lot of people and I do like that. When it is quiet—when it is just me. 'Cause then I can just take my shoes off or play music or things like that and relax instead of having to be 'on' all the time." After school ends, the room is a personal hideaway where she can sit alone with her feet on the table with her shoes off.

And when it is not empty, the room denotes something different to her and her friends, "Then it is also nice when my friends—a lot of the time people will end up gathering in here." To illustrate, she added, "because it is like 'Oh, I was just walking to my classroom and look everyone is just sitting here so I'll join too.' So, everyone is sitting here and chats away. That's fun. And, I can sit in my comfy chair and just be there—not have to participate. I'm going to be tired over here," as she gestures to an imaginary group of friends and telling them, "'You all do that thing.' I still get to be involved but I don't have to do anything to be involved." Her office is a coveted space in the era of open classroom spaces where few teachers in new buildings have a space they can fill with peers or with anything else since most elementary classrooms do not have walls. Penny's room, with a paucity of student seating since she sees one student at a time, has many places for both adults and little people to sit.

Penny's story emphasizes the way the space allows her to be involved and included by proximity and ownership. Her contribution to gatherings can be passive, and this mode of engaging with peers allows her to shift from alert to sleepy without compromising her ability to belong and feel included. This aspect of her story fits with the needs of people with narcolepsy. It also illustrates a goal for employers and managers who work with people who have narcolepsy, which is to enable passive and active ways of creating value. When people with narcolepsy are sleepy, they need to be able to switch to the tasks that require less accuracy and attention to detail; and when they are alert they should be able to engage in the activities that require that mindset.

There are aspects of Penny's job and space that fit her needs as a person with narcolepsy, and there are aspects of teaching that are less flexible. Instead of attempting to evaluate traits and label them as flexible or inflexible, which are relative terms, the idea of congruency and incongruency is more appropriate for addressing the multidimensional work of teaching. An example of an inflexibility and incongruence is Penny's proclivity for walking around her office without shoes and socks. When she goes outside of her office like this, it solicits attention. This is a somewhat benign example of a misfit, or when the wants and needs of a body do not match what a context will provide (Garland-Thomson, 2011). This interpretation section will discuss some of the ways her narcolepsy exists in a context that does not provide opportunities for adaptation or accommodation while also reflecting on the ways Penny has been able to make her space and her narcolepsy fit each other.

Many aspects of Penny's work environment are incongruent with the needs of a person with narcolepsy. As described above, when people pass her window—students, teachers, and administrators—all expect to see her and, as Penny put it, "I have to be awake and doing things." Each moment of her day should be filled with specific activities that she should be able to perform at the specified time. Like her tardiness, when she gets off schedule, everyone knows about it. The service she provides is legally mandated, which means that to get behind schedule, perhaps to finish a lesson or because of a mistake, affects her ability to meet the specified time commitment for other students. As she put it, "I have to see them for that number of minutes" even if sleepiness settles upon her. The schedule demands of working at an elementary school are also difficult for Penny because of the need to drive early in the morning.

Everyone occasionally will get behind, be late, or make mistakes, but it would be a mistake to think of her mistakes as issues everyone deals with. Not only does this perspective undermine the impact of the disability, but in failing to *see* the problem, supervisors in similar situations may also fail to find a solution for someone like Penny in the form of accommodations, help, or schedule changes. During my first interview with Penny, we talked about what she did before deciding to return to school to become a speech pathologist. When reflecting on the difference between working at a theater company and what she does now, the inflexibility of her schedule is a major issue. She observed, "if [I] needed something that was up and active, I would pick that thing off the to-do list. If I wanted to sit and work on something, whereas now I've got to be there by 7:30 [a.m.], and the whole day is scheduled out, and I have to follow that schedule and it's bam, bam, bam, bam all day long and it is exhausting." The rigid schedule of being a speech pathologist teacher for young children seems largely at odds with a health condition that changes her level of alertness from moment to moment.

However, it would be simplistic to suggest that strict scheduling and narcolepsy are always incompatible. Rather, the uncertainty around performance, her unfamiliarity with narcolepsy and issues of accommodation, and her probationary status as a new hire right out of graduate school, all create a context where narcolepsy may potentially mean the end of a career path that recently began. While I certainly hope that this is the least likely way Penny's story will unfold, this potentiality is clear. For example, another participant, Levi, found that working part time, four days a week instead of five, was a manageable way to have narcolepsy and a career in computer science. Sable, on the other hand, found that narcolepsy changed her dreams and her personality. After being awarded disability retirement, Sable tried to pursue her dream of becoming a park ranger by taking jobs that let her work outside. As she told me about this she recalled, "Almost every other job—except for when I was a kid—before the federal government, almost every other job, I've been fired it seems like. And it's saddening. It takes you down." For people like Sable and Jane, who are both either disability retirement or Social Security disability, narcolepsy and full-time employment are wholly incommensurable.

Inattention, Delays, and Mistakes

The main symptoms of narcolepsy are fairly easy to read about and understand in an abstract sense, but from the person's subjective perspective, knowing about one's own sleepiness is significantly more obscure. As Penny and I continued to talk, she explained how one day she had a "narcolepsy type day" in which, "I could barely function I was so tired—falling asleep. If I feel like that's what's causing the issue then yeah. But it doesn't always connect for me. I think sometimes things happen and it doesn't connect," moving her hands rapidly around in front of her face indicating confusion.

I asked, "Hindsight?"

"Yeah. Looking back I guess that was really connected with that although it was sort of," while using her hands to signal a single contained situation.

I chimed in to tell her about a little error I made in writing an email that haunted me. Later, I wrote a poem about it (Eugene, 2017). Penny explained how she simply failed to notice that her license was expired. Then she described how she made a little mistake on a student's report that had big consequences, "We were writing progress report data and I completely missed an entire goal for a kid. Completely missed it. And they were like, 'I go through and write out a list of the entire goals,' 'I did that.' They're like, 'I do this [goal] and this [goal] and that's how I don't.' I was like, 'No, I did all those things. I did everything everyone else is doing. I checked off all the goals and I completely missed that one. Like I have not touched it. I'm sorry.' Oh my god!" At this she laughed lightly.

I paused before adding, "These little mistakes. They don't seem so little when they happen. Like, 'I know I was supposed to do this, but for some reason it wasn't working.'"

To finish my initial thought Penny said, "They have big consequences."

Earlier in the interview I asked about a specific example of how narcolepsy affected her work. She started by sharing that the kids don't notice it, but, "There are definitely times when I get to the end of a session and I have no clue what happened in that session because I was mostly asleep for it, and I was sitting there trying to hide the yawn the whole time. I'm trying to be excited about what I'm doing, but really I'm like, 'What's he doing, what's he doing, great, we're done!' And then I feel bad because they're not getting what they need, or what they deserve." Penny went on to say how she was always trying to balance her tiredness with making sure she gave them good services. For example, if she is not functioning well and is late finishing with one student, then it might not be worth going to get the next one if she is not going to do a good job at squeezing his lesson into a smaller spot. When Penny is struggling with sleepiness she has trouble focusing her eyes because she is so tired.

Inattention is often a form of excessive daytime sleepiness; therefore, a person with narcolepsy can feel perfectly awake but still be prone to making mistakes. The moments of not being able to "take data" that Penny discussed at the beginning of her first interview is an example of inattentional blindness that may be caused by narcolepsy. In addition to inattention there is also a tendency towards hyperactivity in that some people with narcolepsy can be prone to moving on to another task before completing the first one.

As I talked about this, Penny chimed in with an example of this aspect of narcolepsy, "Until I started medication, I couldn't make bacon because it was just long enough for me to get bored and walk away. And then I'd burn it because I'd forget about it. So, I couldn't make it."

She took a breath and continued, "So then I started medication and one day I actually made bacon and I didn't burn it; I was like, 'Oh, my God.

I made the bacon. I did it right! It's edible.' It was always like I would sit there flipping it and flipping it and the next thing you know I'm like 'What is that smell? Oh my god! The bacon!' as I'm halfway across the house doing something else because I just couldn't attend to the bacon. People are like, 'It takes two to three minutes' I'm like 'I can't sit there for three minutes.'" Penny grinned widely and we both started to laugh at the story in a way that showed that perhaps we both felt similarly about it.

While chuckling I said, "That is true. I love that story because yeah, that's the kind of thing that people totally take for granted. Thinking it's easy, 'everybody can do it,' but when your brain has something else in mind. Maybe it's not too easy when that happens." To help with issues of inattention, I rely on my Apple Watch to help me remember big and small plans. Once I've shown her my little helper, she pulled out a small tower that resembles a stop light from behind her computer. It was a Learning Resources time tracker.

With a teacher's cadence she explained, "That's why I got this wonderful timer that I set for twenty minutes because I have twenty-minute sessions. It's fifteen minutes on green and then switches to yellow for three minutes. And then red for two minutes."

Impressed and curious I exclaimed, "That's so cool!"

"I go, 'Okay, this is for the kid so they know.'"

We both broke into laughs, and I clapped in delight.

Still giggling, she continued by adding, "that we work while it's green. And we play when it's yellow and pick up when it's red. It's not for the kids. It's so I know, 'Oh, twenty minutes is up now,' because keeping track of the time was too difficult."

I gushed, "That is so brilliant. I love that." Then I explain how I have had difficulty breaking up college classes into smaller chunks because of what I call an inability to feel time. Not feeling time is the consequence of experiencing inattention where the center of my focus is the only thing my brain is processing. In short, I had to devote a significant part of my mental attention to thinking about time because of inattention.

She reiterated, "It's not for the kids. It's so I know, 'Oh twenty minutes is up now' because keeping track of the time was too difficult."

Referring to my Apple Watch, I submitted that I might be able to get it to help me with feeling time.

Penny added, "I've even set this for if I need to make sure I go home on time. Because I get lost in things."

"Exactly, you are totally not alone there."

The idea that someone might not "feel time" was something that I experienced regularly, and it is an example of a nonexperience that comes to have a name and meaning when in conversation with others who are wrestling with the same problems. I was invigorated by this part of our conversation. Over the next few days, I told many people, including my mentor, about the timer and the discovery of this way to talk about my inability to feel time. I quickly learned how to silence my watch and have since used it several times to help me feel time—through the haptic pulses it makes when an alarm goes off. Since this conversation, I have used this language to discuss and think about what my brain is able to do and what it at times is unable to do. Together Penny and I created or discovered a phrase and it is an artifact we can share as people who needed novel words to discuss the experiences associated with having narcolepsy.

Both Penny and I worked in environments that encouraged or required us to break every encounter with students into smaller components and to be able to do this temporal arithmetic with little or no effort. Not being able to feel time also marks our brains as neurodiverse by not moralizing the trait the way that phrases like "loses track of time" or "flow" create negative and positive intonations. This conversation moves past the exchange of messages and transforms possibilities because we have created something together and the idea we have created has a substance we both recognize as valid.

In addition to experiencing issues with inattention, inattentional blindness and memory problems are a part of the brain fog of excessive daytime sleepiness. In *Consciousness and the Brain*, Stanislas Dehaene (2014) introduces the concept of inattentional blindness by describing how, "Avid readers, concentrated chess players, and focused mathematicians know all too well that intellectual absorption can create long periods of mental isolation, during which we lose all awareness of our surroundings" (p. 34). He then goes on to describe Dan Simons and Christopher Charis's (2010) experiment known as "the invisible gorilla,"[1] which is a film that features two teams passing a basketball back and forth. When viewers are asked to keep their eyes on one team they are often oblivious to the gorillas that come into the room. This act of focusing causes the person in a gorilla costume in the center of the film to vanish. There are invisible gorillas littered throughout the day of someone experiencing excessive daytime sleepiness. Penny's account of not being able to "take data" refers to how when she is teaching a lesson she should be able to make note of whether the student is listening and responding to her explanations in a way that shows they understand or are confused. She was not able to collect this type of data because it was the invisible gorilla and her brain was focused on delivering content. I recognized what she was describing because I suspected that maybe something like this would happen to me. Not being able to take a moment to check to see if students are bored, are not taking notes, are disinterested, or are distracted meant not being able to react and adjust my lesson plans on the spot. My not being treated for disrupted sleep likely accounted for our shared experiences. As my nighttime sleep improved, this issue became less significant.

Immediately following the second interview with Penny, I continued to mold a description of inattentional blindness and used a metaphor to describe it. Many people are familiar with the idea that phone numbers have seven digits because it was believed that people can remember up to seven pieces of information at a single moment. The actual way attention and memory works is significantly more complicated, but for the sake of the metaphor let us use the number seven. Now to visualize this concept, imagine that you have seven TV screens in your brain—each one represents a piece of information that a brain can process at a given moment. Line them up like the rows of TVs seen in electronics stores. At any given moment, for most people there are different details on each screen. For example, one screen is on grammar, one is on the main idea, one is on typing, another on time, and so on. Inattention means not having seven screens but instead having only three or four screens. Fewer screens means someone is making decisions based on less information and engaging fewer tasks in everyday life. It means, while typing an email, losing track of the beginning of the sentence by the time you get to the end of it because there were not enough screens to remember it. Again, this is an extreme version of what may happen to nearly everyone in any given moment. At any given time, there are a number of things that remain outside of our sphere of awareness until they are called upon or are felt. For example, the feel of our clothes on our skin enters our perception in this way, because unless we think of it the sensation stays below our conscious awareness. Inattention is a circumscription of what is perceivable.

Inattentional blindness is not all big scary animals, elementary aged or costumed. From the perspective of neurodiversity, it is also an asset. I attribute part of my insatiable appetite for books, paper and audio, to my enhanced capacity to be immersed into the world of the author. Doing long stretches of reading and writing is also amicable to inattentional blindness that makes distractions and restlessness less likely. The benefits are that when you only have four or three screens you pay more attention to those fewer screens. Their details and nuances are more apparent and they offer a richer sense of understanding. Penny's experience of mistakes and inattention was addressed by identifying what her brain was having difficulty doing and then finding a way to compensate for it.

Several participants admitted to having similar issues with concentration, performance, and memory while working. John, for example said that he decided to try sodium oxybate (Xyrem) because:

> My life was falling apart about to lose—I could have potentially lost my job because I really couldn't focus at all. I was all over the place every day. I'd sit in my office reading through Google News articles and jumping from anything on the internet that looked interesting and then doing work.

However, it took three years to find the right balance between the Xyrem, his sleep apnea treatment, and the right stimulant. He noticed how certain stimulants would turn him into a monotone speaker, and as a person that does a lot of speaking as a self-employed director of an addiction treatment center, he needed to be an effective public speaker. When people with narcolepsy get together there tends to be a lot of talk about medications. Medication talk, like talk about symptoms, is a way of bridging the individual meaning the medication has for the individual with the role it plays in the lives of others. Medication changes and adjustments are major fixtures in the landscape of people with narcolepsy, and it is only with the help of medication they are able to excel at work. The need to talk about this part of narcolepsy is shared by people who have gone through it or are in the middle of the search to find the right drugs to let them have a sense of normality and alertness. Medication is also the key to passing as not disabled in a world where few people understand what narcolepsy means and fewer who would welcome unscheduled naps at work. Penny found support in the friendship of a person who lets her nap in a room that does not broadcast her sleep to the school. She also found it in the way her room facilitated a socializing without her having to do the socializing.

WORKING HARDER WITH LESS

This chapter highlights the juxtaposition of the crucial life-sustaining activity of work and a condition that interferes with a person's capacity to stay awake during the day. For some, these two aspects of everyday life constantly conflict while others have more amicable employers or manageable symptoms. In addition to sharing the stories of participants, I have also shared insights into my own lived experiences of working with narcolepsy. Accordingly, personal head notes and archival materials have been interwoven here to illustrate the work of writing, researching, interviewing, and teaching while managing a condition that is characterized by numerous unscheduled romps in la la land or what is otherwise known as excessive daytime sleepiness.

To grapple with the oxymoronic concept of working while sleepy or while allowing for unscheduled naps and breaks, one must first discuss the way people with narcolepsy must do more to do less. I am referring to the extra work of managing narcolepsy that occurs at home and at work that nevertheless recognizes the inevitability of sleepiness, inefficiency, and errors. This leads to more work in the form of double checking one's work or allowing for more time and putting in more effort in general. This extra time spent working may or may not be compensated. There are other ways people with narcolepsy manage to be productive and valued employees, as Grouse's story describes.

Grouse, who is a librarian at a Columbus area university, described his practice of making time for narcolepsy when he stated, "It can be things sort of like the feast and famine phenomena where there are stretches where I lag and struggle and just can't focus and just can't get stuff done, and then there are stretches where I can sort of buckle down and go like gangbusters for a while and sort of make it up. There are episodes during the year where I have to do certain things during the period of the year, like the spring, managing budgets and things like that, where I have to do it. I just have to force myself to do it. I just have to like brute, brute, you know."

I offered, "Yeah, force."

He clarified, "determination to do it." Then he went on and said, "To do certain things but there are other times where I slack off so it evens out. It evens out but it is very inconsistent, very up and down." I liked this description, feast and famine, because it fits some of my working patterns in terms of the deluge of work that flows towards deadlines and awaits the end of each semester.

Penny's account highlights how she was given a rigid schedule with every moment of her day planned out, but little by little she changed this schedule and the expectation that she will operate in a predictable manner. She related, "I feel like all the teachers have learned that I don't follow my schedule, and they finally just like accept that I send them the schedule and that's not like, like I don't even look at it anymore." She went on to explain how they know that the schedule is really more of a wish list than a plan, "we all know like I'm not following it." The inflexibility of the schedule Penny must provide to teachers is balanced out by the way people are willing to change their expectations. Like Penny's coworkers, changing preconceptions about sleep and productivity is key to understanding and appreciating people with narcolepsy as productive people who have valuable contributions to make.

Penny was reticent about requesting work accommodations, especially since she is still learning what narcolepsy means personally and for her career. All my interviewees who were employed seemed equally committed to working. While the issue of Social Security disability came up occasionally in my interviews, it was not something that any of the interviewees seemed interested in. All were making sacrifices to improve their performance at work and saw how narcolepsy was affecting their ability to meet expectations in terms of performance and tardiness. Some of my interviewees shared their condition with their employer and had supportive resources that allowed for naps during the day, while others did not tell employers or were self-employed. Family life, home, friendships, hobbies, entertainment, and fitness were often abandoned or minimized because of the sense that alertness and energy should be reserved for their jobs. For many of the people I interviewed, work became life to the detriment of family, friends, hobbies, and other fulfilling activities. The exceptions to this were Levi and Aurora who each had activities they committed to outside of work. Penny described how she could not invite a friend over who was an incredibly neat person because of how many chores are left undone at home. Work is perceived as being worth all the sacrifices she makes to ensure she has energy for it and does her absolute best. At times, the configuration of my life also attested to the lengths people may go to continue working by cutting out or down other parts of life. Grouse, for example, describes himself as "extremely socially isolated." And in listening to his story this was never something he pursued, rather it was forced upon him by the overwhelming experience of exhaustion that accompanied efforts to socialize at work-related social events. Many people with narcolepsy pour themselves into work, while perhaps unfortunately or perhaps fortunately, few may bear witness to this unique form of heroism.

There are three types of narcoleptic employees: the undiagnosed narcoleptics, the ones that have most symptoms under control, and those who are still working with doctors to find the right medications for their condition. While Penny's story includes accounts from her undiagnosed status, for the most part I am concerned with the latter two types of employees with narcolepsy. Employers and educators should be aware that the period of working to find the right medicine can take a year or several years, during which time performance may be affected by excessive daytime sleepiness and other symptoms. Meanwhile the employee will likely put a great deal of energy and effort into doing the best they can and still fall short—all while developing grit and a habit of working harder than their peers. Even so, these traits eventually will make them an asset once the condition is better managed. In short, while errors and mistakes need not be tolerated, they can likely be easily accommodated by providing extra time and extra flexibility. This is the ideal scenario for people who are diagnosed with narcolepsy. Elaine experienced this type of unequivocal support and accommodation from her employer, while the rest of my interviewees and myself face various attitudes about narcolepsy and accommodation measures that are less than ideal.

In writing about the productivity of people with narcolepsy, I must look directly upon the ugly fragility of human understanding. Many people labor to create a sense of reality in which being wrong is a trait of Others, enemies, and the evil—and rarely a personal trait. There is no shortage of leaders who eagerly demonstrate this tendency to disown the possibility of being wrong. However, history attests to all the things people were wrong about, while often keeping the evanescent structures that nurtured these wrong ideas safely tucked away and out of sight. This orientation towards the past allows us to similarly embrace today naively oblivious to the innumerable ways much of what is certain may also be crushingly wrong, and as time moves forward people will someday again spend their evenings being amused by the beautiful wrongness of today. This declaration is a prelude to acknowledging the unequivocal wrongness of how narcolepsy is often viewed by others. Yet, as a person living with narcolepsy and studying it, the chimerical nature of its wrongness galvanizes me to chase it.

For the moment, let us put aside the amoral lenses of disability studies and physiopathology to explore what may be wrong with narcolepsy. Is it simply a breach in social norms and expectations, as Wolf-Meyer (2012) suggests? For the sake of debate, let us suppose that it is a riddle: there is everything wrong with narcolepsy and yet nothing is wrong with those who live with it. Is it the sleep or the social absence that debases their position as people who are capable of error? Is it the way the perceptual wall of sleep intrudes while participating in an exchange of employer and employee, or between teacher and student? While the exact nature of the breach may be chimerical the material consequences of having narcolepsy are less obscure. For Penny and others, their errors and mistakes are a clear demonstration of what the adult world often disapproves of. This struggle to reconcile the value-producing activity of work and the value-draining persistence of unawareness is at the center of understanding the narcoleptic in a workplace or anyplace where mistakes are often unwelcome.

The task of this chapter, and the task of the book, is to reveal how, for people with narcolepsy and similar conditions, value and unawareness coexist in everyday negotiations and can be seen in narratives of the unending work of living in a world that is often organized around the idea that the two are incommensurable. How can a person go moment to moment sliding into and out of sleep and sleepiness all the while caring for children, working, driving, loving, and celebrating life? What keeps them from falling into a hole within themselves, and what ideas reach into that hole time and again to pull them out? This is the fundamental tension that this research attends to, and by attending to it aspires to enlighten those who might otherwise misunderstand or erase narcoleptics.

Let me now update the idea that there is something wrong with narcolepsy or narcoleptics by instead framing narcolepsy as a type of neurodiversity. To approach narcolepsy as a neurodiversity means that instead of focusing on the deficits people experience, one instead recognizes the different ways their brain functions to acknowledge both strengths and weaknesses. By describing the subjective experience of someone who will drift between different states of alertness and sleepiness throughout the day, I highlight how this difference has both horror and novelty. Medicine frequently has a big role to play in helping people with narcolepsy manage their sleep and alertness, but it is unable to completely excise all symptoms of narcolepsy with surgical precision.

People with narcolepsy, idiopathic hypersomnia, or other fatigue-inducing conditions may experience sleep and wakefulness in terms that are vastly different from people without such a condition. One of the first major obstacles for people with narcolepsy involves challenges around communicating about the condition and about what it means for work. Some people, like John, will give up on talking about narcolepsy to their family members; while others, like Penny, will celebrate the hard-won recognition of the physiological experience of narcolepsy. Months after our interview I learned from Penny that once her medicine started to improve her level of energy, her husband started to recognize the validity of her condition. A year after our interview Penny explained that her husband not only changed, but he apologized for having called her "lazy." He now comes to her defense quickly when he thinks that Penny is being too hard on herself.

Describing narcolepsy as a form of neurodiversity means recognizing that people with narcolepsy are different from many people in fundamental ways. One of the benefits of the neurodiversity framework is it reduces the need to understand the pathophysiology of narcolepsy and lets me and others focus on everyday issues of strategies and techniques. For Penny, and the others I have interviewed, much of the work of managing narcolepsy is left to the individual. Consequently, this work is hidden and remains unacknowledged except by the few people they may talk to. These confidantes often are people who live with narcoleptics at home or are otherwise intimately involved in their everyday lives. The next chapter explores what narcolepsy symptoms may come to mean at home.

NOTE

1. Their Invisible Gorilla website includes the original video, demonstrations, and other videos from their research and information about their book. Simons and Charis (2010) refers to the behavior as selective attention instead of inattentional blindness. Both terms have troubling implications in discussions of disability.

Chapter 4

At Home with Narcolepsy

Home is an expansive concept that encompasses both places and processes that range from a grandparent's house, a customized van, a tent under a bridge underpass, a mortgaged house in a suburb, a shared apartment with chosen kin, or a distant spot on a map. In a country where the percentage of adults who are single is rising from year to year, the meaning of home is likely to continue to shift in tandem with continuing environmental, economic, social, and political transformations. Before exploring how narcolepsy takes shape in a home, I will briefly survey the idea of home as a site of intimate meaning making in social and cultural research.

One's childhood home and one's adult home can be both a dynamic symbolic concept and a physical place characterized by intimate familial and nonfamilial relations. The COVID-19 pandemic radically shifted the meaning of home and the nature of the work that occurred there. Prior to the pandemic, for some social theorists, home was a site of social reproduction where raising children and requisite preparation for work took place. Although much of this was unpaid labor, when it was done by paid labor it was often done by marginalized or disadvantaged women (Cockayne, 2021). The shifts the pandemic brought about varied across the social differences that stratify the lived experience of being at home across lines of race, economic class, gender, sexuality, and age (Cockayne, 2021). For example, a meta study that examined eleven research papers published in 2021 and 2022 about homeschooling during the pandemic found that for students with special education needs, the switch to homeschooling had negative consequences for the parents and the students (Dobosz et al., 2023). Furthermore, in a qualitative study in the Netherlands, mothers of children with intellectual disabilities decided to bring their child home from the residential facility that took care of them because of a number of reasons, such as "doing what was best for them, providing protection and not wanting to be separated from their offspring" (Vereijken et al., 2022, p. 156). Once home, parents had to, once again, strike a balance between supporting their children and their own wants or hopes for the future.

Of course, Black feminists have long challenged the public/private dualism that often characterizes discourse about home (Collins, 1986). Cultural critic and feminist, bell hooks (1997), wrote passionately about how home was a place where her opinions and voice was not appreciated consequently galvanizing her to *talk back* to those who sought to silence her via her prolific writings. Home may or may not be the basis of one's supportive network that provides messages of reassurance, validation, and acceptance while also sharing valued resources. While many may be tempted to discuss family communication as a source of social support, family can also be a source of deeply invalidating messages that spur individuals to seek out more nurturing relationships (Adams, 2006; Nero, 2016). The relational dynamics that may be core to a hegemonic understanding of home, and the material domesticity that may accompany it, is not a universal ideal despite the existence of discourses and businesses that profit from propagating images and stories of home as a symbol of happiness, security, and belonging (Presswood, 2020). Furthermore, there are myriad intricacies involved in the way that performances of being home or not being home bare on one's identity and sense of self for transnational persons (Chawla, 2014). Any brief exploration of the concept of home will have many inevitable lacunae because underneath the shifting and multilayered nature of home are multitudes of vulnerable people with an unsatiated need for nurturing, care, and comfort despite all that a home may create or symbolize.

Within health communication research, home may be a site of caregiving, birthing, social support, and coping (Broderick, 2016; Doshi, 2014). In the area of communicating to manage health, home is also a context where health information behaviors can occur. For example, when passively encountering health information about type 2 diabetes, participants who were at home were more likely to share this information with others than when they actively sought information or were not at home (Broekhuis et al., 2022). This reflects the way that home is a place where people may often willingly influence one another. Within a socio-ecological model, home is a part of the interpersonal level of social factors that impact health behaviors like what someone decided had for lunch today (Baiocchi-Wagner, 2011). Home has the potential to play a range of roles in a person's life and health.

My very first interview for this project was with Cameron who was twenty-seven and was diagnosed five years earlier. She discussed how her life was compressed by unexpected naps because she found that narcolepsy made seemingly simple tasks somewhat unwieldy. While Cameron and I initially agreed to meet at her home, when she canceled the second interview, I was sympathetic—her life seemed incredibly busy and the time she had for it was choked by sleepiness, tiredness, and unfinished tasks. If her home was a place of mounting tension and unfinished housework, I had begun to wonder if other interviewees may also be reticent about inviting me home for an interview. Her predicament also demonstrates why interviewing at home became unlikely and rare as I continued my interviews. What follows is an intimate portrait of narcolepsy at home through the insights gleaned in my interview with Elaine.

My directions took me into a rural area where I drove down a type of road whose unfamiliarity eluded me at first—unlike the Appalachian hilly roads that wind up and down the college town of Athens, this road ran straight for miles. The flat midwestern road was surrounded by fields of mowed grass and lush spring trees. I quickly looked around to see if someone might be looking at me before reaching for my smartphone. Balancing the phone over the steering wheel, the camera captured this empty stretch while also capturing a piece of what I felt when I first saw it (see cover).

About five minutes later, I parked outside of a colonial-style two-story house painted a silvery gray with bright white trim. Across the street from the house are acres of golden grass and another long straight road that flowed into a rural horizon. A little boy met me at the door and his mom encouraged him to show me the way through the house. Elaine was holding a baby not too far in front of him. On the inside, I saw and sniffed the rich mahogany or pine accents of the recently renovated home. She told me that they were trying to put something together. My interest piqued when I saw something vaguely familiar. Elaine explained that she was trying to put together a tent for them. Putting my purse down, I recalled the tent/house I helped put together for my nieces and nephew in Houston last Christmas. This must be what they were working on when I arrived.

Elaine put her baby, who I will call Joy, in a bouncer that hung from the doorway between the dining area and the family room. Joy bounced there happily smiling while giggling and squealing. She had the most adorable bright eyes. We had put together a few sections of the round plastic parts of the frame when her son, who I will call Dale, discovered it and then endeavored to take it all apart. Eventually I asked, "So, how do you want to do this?" referring to the interview. I was willing to do it in the family room, before I noticed that her one-year-old, whom Elaine had taken out of the bouncer, was constantly moving to various parts of the room—a moment earlier we turned to see Dale grab my purse, which was sitting on the couch. He was about to dump the contents out to see what was inside. Meanwhile, we spent a few minutes on the tent before Elaine began to suspect that we were missing a central piece. Dale must have hidden it or dropped it someplace. Elaine explained what it looked like, and I immediately saw that this would explain the difficulty we were having in making it ready for the next step. We soon abandoned the structure to be taken apart by Dale, and she showed me her kitchen table where we talked for the next seventy-two minutes.

This chaotic introduction to Elaine's world—trying to build something together and failing together—all while not breaking a sweat is an adept metaphor for life with narcolepsy. It is also a metaphor for what it means to have narcolepsy in a house with two young children. Moving forward, this chapter will introduce Elaine and her life with narcolepsy followed by an analysis of what being at home with narcolepsy means based on the analysis of my interview with Elaine. The themes that emerged reveal that Elaine's sleepiness tends to be unpredictable and misunderstood which has implications on the roles Elaine fills while at home. Unlike the rest of the interviewees who were highlighted in the chapters about working, driving, and being active with narcolepsy, Elaine was only available for one interview because of the roles she was constantly juggling as a working mother with young children. Despite the drawbacks of not having had two opportunities to talk with her, what she shared is nevertheless compelling, illustrative, and insightful.

ELAINE'S DIAGNOSIS STORY

I met Elaine at the May gathering of the support group meeting in Columbus. She came in a few minutes late with a young baby tied to her with a toddling toddler and a husband in tow. After a few minutes of the meeting, he took the curious toddler out to walk around the restaurant. We all were envious of Elaine when she chimed in to tell us about how her employers let her take naps and were eager to provide other accommodations. At thirty-five, she was diagnosed with narcolepsy without cataplexy earlier this year, but she thinks her symptoms started to show up at the age of sixteen or seventeen. Although classrooms are a place where she often falls asleep, she has a four-year degree and lives out in Lancaster, Ohio, but she grew up in Pickerington where her high school yearbook gave her the superlative of "class sleeper."

Even though she was called "class sleeper," her symptoms were limited to predictable places, and like many people with narcolepsy, she became accustomed to falling asleep in class, while driving, and while watching TV or movies. To adjust, she made sure she had a short commute that was less than fifteen minutes, adding, "But honestly, I guess I kinda thought that everybody fell asleep when they drove. Like, I didn't realize how abnormal it is, I guess. You know, falling asleep at lectures." After she ran off the road a couple of times, she mentioned it to a couple people at work who said, "'That's not normal. You need to go to the doctor to get it checked out. You can't be running off the road every day you drive.'" Elaine had begun falling asleep like this daily. Her pregnancies were initially a barrier to the normal diagnosis process because the altered sleep of pregnant women impacts the results of the sleep test. During her second pregnancy her doctors decided to go ahead and do a sleep test, and as they suspected, the test turned out to be inconclusive. After Joy was born—four months ago—she went to the doctor and had the sleep study where she was diagnosed with narcolepsy without cataplexy.

This diagnosis story is unique in that her coworkers intervened and not someone closer to her who might have noticed her sleepiness. Yet this is another example of how people with narcolepsy come to better understand narcolepsy through interactions with others. The nature of sleepiness and sleep itself suppresses self-awareness and cognitive activity, and hence in our ability to recognize a problem may easily be impeded by the very nature of the condition (Naumann et al., 2006; Zamarian et al., 2014). This is in addition to the long onset of symptoms that allow people with narcolepsy to grow more and more sleepy over the course of years, subsequently finding sleepiness to be a familiar and expected experience. However, as her story shows, this form of sleepiness and sleep will eventually, in most times, butt up against a world that has different norms around sleep and sleepiness. Delayed recognition is a common feature of narcolepsy diagnosis stories because often it is only through failing to meet unspoken expectations around sleep and wakefulness that peoplerealize the possibility of an underlying medical condition.

Elaine's narrative illustrates what it can mean to have narcolepsy at home. Although only when the interview occurred, two distinct stories emerged—one is the story of working while narcoleptic, and the other is the story of being a mother of young children while figuring out what narcolepsy means for her life and her family. This chapter will focus on the latter story but also recognizes that her understanding of what her home affords her is based on comparisons to what her work setting affords. For Elaine, experiencing narcolepsy at home entails moments of fulfillment and moments of discontent. In addition to focusing on Elaine's story I will also share some of the stories from other participants about dealing with narcolepsy at home.

For many of the people I interviewed, home was simultaneously a site of tension and a reprieve from being at work where narcolepsy can impair productivity in ways that are difficult to explain much less compensate for. To explore the ways a person with narcolepsy is a misfit in their own homes is to explore how narcolepsy may impair everyday life and intimate relationships bringing about both moments of fulfillment and moments of discontent. Elaine has a sense of control at home that she cannot find at work. However, work offers a type of empathy absent from her relationships with her husband and mother who compose Elaine's personal support system. Lastly, this chapter will present stories of being at home with narcolepsy from other interviewees to explore the themes of discontent and fulfillment.

For many people, home is a place of relaxation and comfort; but for many people with hidden disabilities, home is also a site where the intense and indispensable backstage work of managing a chronic condition occurs. Bodies inhabit and engage spaces differently, and this means that what one's home affords reflects a person's perceived capacities. This research project brought me to many different homes, some were quaint and worry-free, while others were homes where tension and disorder suggested orderings that may be difficult to decipher at a glance. Each home suggested a different configuration of layered relationships between bodies and space. More unforeseen than the wide range of adjustments and fits was the reticence many clearly expressed about inviting me to their home. As discussed in chapter 2, I grew up in a household that was often not presentable to strangers most days of the week; and in the months following my time in the field while juggling new medications, engaging in a job hunt, and preparing for classes, my apartment came undone in new and frightening ways. This most intimate of spaces, like every space, allows narcoleptics activities in accordance with our capacities.

AT HOME WITH UNPREDICTABLE AND MISUNDERSTOOD SLEEPINESS

As I discussed aspects of my methodology, which is covered in the appendix, the baby in her arms started to wail. Elaine began to pat her on the back as I confirmed their contact information. The baby—an infant who had visibly grown since the day I first saw her at the support group meeting—stopped crying as her back was patted. Instead of having Elaine fill out the demographic form, I filled it in so she could continue to pat her infant to sleep. Joy fell asleep about forty minutes into the interview.

When I asked about her medications, our conversation somewhat switched from pre-interview to interview as she sighed and said, "You see, that's what we are still trying to figure out."

Her baby whimpered at the changed pace and tone in her voice. She explained how the issue of medication was tied up with how long she was going to breastfeed, and now that she is done breastfeeding they have to find out what medications she will be on to manage her symptoms. A children's TV show played in the background for the older boy. For a few minutes, it sounded like he was determined to put the tent together on his own. Dale did not go into the other room until Elaine got up and closed the toy box beside our table. She told him, "Stay out of there," as I discussed the last bit of paperwork she needed to do.

After telling me about how her coworkers told her to go to the doctor to see why she was so sleepy, she abruptly pivoted and said, "And I started falling asleep with patients, like while I was cleaning teeth—while I was like doing the micro sleep thing. Nobody ever noticed that I was falling asleep but I was definitely falling asleep."

To better understand what she was describing, I asked what microsleep is like for her.

"I just start kind of dozing as I'm working, just repeatedly though. Not ever really nodding off completely, I don't think. Well, I mean, I do because I'm doing things I don't really remember doing it." She works as a dental assistant, and as she confided this images flashed in my mind's eye of the danger she might be putting herself and others in.

Then I added, "That's something else, I can't remember what it is called, but that is, um, automatic behavior." As discussed in chapter 2, automatic behavior is a symptom of narcolepsy in which persons drift off while doing a familiar repetitive task that has been done several times before. These lapses are perceived as a loss of awareness or consciousness, experiencing a blank moment and some people have reported being partially aware of their automatic behavior during the act (Morandin & Bruck, 2013).

To which she responded, "Oh yeah!"

To make sure she understood, I stated, "Automatic behavior, because you're present but because it is something you've done in the past your self-awareness can check out and you're like, suddenly you're here. It's like, 'Where have you been?'" hoping she was familiar with the concept. She was not falling asleep in the conventional sense of the concept—few intrusions of sleep into wake states are similar to conventional experiences of sleep. Rather she was sleepy and experienced automatic behavior, but this correction does little to ease the sense of alarm her confession brought. Of course, this might have been an attempt to put myself more at ease at her story.

At this point, Dale brings his sippy cup and sits it on the table and timidly declared, "All gone." Elaine asked him if he wants more but he only repeated himself.

She continued to explain that she does not think her head nods while dozing off because then patients would have noticed and said something. Elaine is describing a sensation that she knows something is happening and is looking for clues to help her understand what it is because her ability to understand her experience of narcolepsy is impinged by the nature of narcolepsy and is further hampered by her unfamiliarity with the condition.

I am familiar with the sense of wondering what happened after experiencing an unexpected symptom. When driving, for example, I could feel a micro sleep happen only through the sensation of waking up that hits me. Otherwise, I explained, there is no evidence of sleep, "because you're still pressing on the gas." This is another example of how narcoleptics' experience of sleep is partial and often bearing little resemblance to nondisordered sleep.

She concurred, "right, yeah. That's kinda how it is for me too. I don't really know that I'm falling asleep until I'm coming back, but I'm presuming it's really quickly; it's not happening for very long."

Our attempt to talk about what happens when our brains are half asleep is one of the reasons why people with narcolepsy benefit from support groups, Facebook groups, more communicative doctors, and may do a lot of information-seeking behaviors—significant portions of the experience of narcolepsy sit right beyond the curtain of consciousness. Our inability to access much less know what is happening is something we can only sometimes admit to ourselves, and then once we do, we are uniquely vulnerable because these fragments of nonmoments are central to what it means to have narcolepsy. Early in our interview and throughout it we worked to put our fragments together to learn how to tell our own stories more fully.

Early in the interview, Elaine used silence to invite me to say more about my experiences with similar symptoms. This request assuaged the occasional guilt I felt about using speaking time during our conversations. Her insistence on hearing my story suggested that she appreciated it and perhaps needed help making sense of what she was experiencing. There were many moments when we finished each other's sentences, and at the end of the interview I suspected that perhaps she needed my stories about narcolepsy just as much if not more than I needed hers.

Control and Support at Home

Elaine's ability to manage moments of unpredictable sleepiness at home became evident once she put it in contrast to her experiences at work where, despite the generous accommodations, she feels unable to control the environment. Elaine shared that her kids are unaware of her sleepiness and naps at this age. She went on to explain how she had her mom help her drive to the two appointments she had one day. Gesturing with her chin to where Dale is watching TV, Elaine explained, "The mornings I don't worry about as much because I generally do fine with my meds in the morning. The afternoon I was pretty worried about after we ate lunch I put—my go-to is *Peppa Pig* because he loves it and he'll sit still for the twenty minutes when it's on or whatever. [Joy] had just eaten and was asleep. I just turned it on and made sure the gates were up and went down and slept for like ten minutes but it was enough to, you know, make me able to drive there and back." Later she added, "I feel like I keep up fine here. It's work where I feel like I can't." She suspected that she should be more active with her husband but otherwise she feels like she is able to do all the housework that should be done. Elaine's experience of narcolepsy at home includes strategies that allow her to control her environment and the demands she responds to. This sense of agency and control is what is missing from her experiences at work.

As an example of how narcolepsy leads to a sense of "sinking," she returned to the topic of her work and explained, "Some days are fine. Some days I feel like I can't keep up. Like I'm just sinking. And patients are scheduled every fifteen minutes and I'm like twenty minutes behind because I just can't, I can't keep up. I can't process. Sometimes I feel like I can't communicate with them well some days." Later in the interview she described being in tears because she was not able to keep up. This struggle to perform at home and at work became a key theme early in her interview. As she went on to tell me more about her life at home and the relationship with her husband, I came to understand that her fear of being discontented lies in the way her desire to be competent at work is based on her desire to financially contribute to her family.

Elaine also is satisfied with the type of help she gets at home from others. I asked, "Do you think there are other relationships that help you manage . . . "

Before I finished my question, she responded, "My mom; she drives me. Whenever I have appointments up at Children's [Hospital] or I have appointments up in Columbus she's usually the one that's driving me around." In sensing an opening and asked about the house by prompting, "tell me a little more about this place because, you know, you talked a little bit about lifestyle adjustments, right, and the commute sounds sleepy, right? You're also not in walking distance to anything, right? . . . Or does this particular home have a particular story?"

After a pause, she explained that she is from Pickerington and her mom lives seven minutes away and, before the kids, they used to live closer to where she works—now they are forty-five minutes away. They decided to move out near her mom to get help with the babies.

Her son returned to the table and said, "All done."

She explained, "We kinda wanted to be closer to family for the help so . . . We just wanted to get back down this way to be closer to family." They have been in the house less than two years. While she is a little less than satisfied with the support her husband offers around the house, Elaine maintains that narcolepsy is not a source of tension between them.

At work, there was a coworker who has dismissed narcolepsy and continued to antagonize Elaine. I asked if she ever joked about narcolepsy, and she said she does not and that it "sucks." She went on to tell me about a coworker who, "I think she thought it was funny and thought that I was just a lazy piece of crap, probably. She would just make comments like, like I mentioned, you know, some people end up on disability because of it or whatever and she's like 'For narcolepsy?' And I'm like, 'You have no idea how terrible this is.'"

Then Elaine continued on to talk about how she went to a continuing education course that took place in Las Vegas, and, "Of all people she was the one sitting next to me through the lecture. I mean, I drank so much coffee I was sick to my stomach and I could not stay awake. I could not stay awake. And she's like, 'What is your problem?'" I interjected, "Oh, and then since it is Vegas, people presume like it's because of a hangover." This type of dismissal and invalidation is more disconfirming than any apathy she may experience at home.

Her inability to change the mind of her coworker allows her to appreciate the agency she has at home around helping her husband understand narcolepsy. As she explained it, she would get "irritated with him because he doesn't get that, you know, I need to be in bed on time. 'You can stay up until 1 and get up at 7 or 6 or whatever, I can't do it.' Like, 'I need you to understand.' But we don't really argue or fight." Although her efforts at educating him have, thus far, failed, his reaction does not seem to dismiss or invalidate her the way her coworker does.

I hummed in agreement and asked, "What do you think he understands about it?"

Elaine described leaving him paperwork for him to read to ensure he knows about it. To clarify she added, "He's not a very empathetic kind of person. If it's not affecting him he doesn't really get it. Like, and he knows that." At this I explained that, as a single woman, I noticed that some men are good at taking on a caregiver role while other guys seem completely unable to take on a caregiver role.

To this she says, "Yeah, my husband is not the caretaker role [type]."

Elaine's busy life with two babies was recently made even more hectic with the diagnosis of narcolepsy symptoms. When I interviewed her, Elaine was in the beginning stages of learning what narcolepsy means to her life and her family. While the people at work are very supportive of her pregnancies and her narcolepsy, she is not able to control the environment there the way she can control it at home. The unpredictable nature of narcolepsy can be better managed at home where she can quickly adapt to what she and her family need.

Other interviewees spoke about the tensions that narcolepsy creates at home. To support and nuance the meaning of narcolepsy at home I will put their stories in conversation with Elaine's story. As previously discussed, many people I spoke with felt that their time at home was often wasted leaving an ever-expanding list of doing the things they hoped to accomplish. When I asked Penny about what she would do if she did not have to work, she explained, "Making my home into a place that I felt proud to show people." However, at the time her husband was convinced that she did not want to do anything. Because of the lack of energy and sleepiness, her husband does a lot of the tasks around the house. As she puts it, "Chores, bills, like any sort of like household thing that needs to happen, he does everything. Taking care of the pets, um yeah everything. Grocery shopping, cooking, cleaning. I help out a little bit but it's a negligible amount." The energy medication provided often was spent pursuing gainful employment to the detriment of the relationships and spaces that comprise a home.

During my first interview with Cynthia, who has lived several years with narcolepsy, she discussed tensions narcolepsy created at home. Before Cynthia's narcolepsy worsened to the point of needing medication, her home life was imperfect, but her sleepiness made dealing with larger issues more difficult. She explained how once her mother passed away, thirteen years ago, she inherited all of her belongings, therefore she moved these things into her own home to work on decluttering in her free time. However, as she put it:

> I keep procrastinating and putting it aside. And so that's kind of how I feel here is like I probably put a lot of things off sometimes. Like I said, I tend to focus more on work, my personal life, and my home life, and all of that suffers because I can't focus on all of these things and get all of these things done. I can only focus on one.

Sleepiness comes in many forms and Cynthia is describing the way inattention, disorganization, and other forms of sleepiness may interfere with being able to take on and complete personal projects. Cynthia's and Penny's accounts are a point of contrast to Elaine's sense of support and control exposing how varied narcolepsy may be when dealing with analogous spaces.

The Misunderstood Sleepy Self

Elaine's account of narcolepsy includes several instances in which she expresses discontent with herself and her sleepiness. Managing her narcolepsy competes for her time, and when that happens she is hesitant to make time for sleep, as she explained, "Napping during the day can't really happen anymore. Or I guess it could but I got to get stuff done around here, you know."

I asked which areas of her life are most affected by narcolepsy.

"Well, my husband ends up having to pick up a lot of the work I can't—mostly on the evenings that I have to work the next day. I go to bed and the house is just a wreck."

Elaine said, "I've never been one that likes to ask people for help. Like I hate to have to ask for help," adding, "I guess I'm too independent or proud." Unlike women more eager to call on partners for a helping hand, Elaine says she has told her husband, "no, I'll do it myself." She continued, "I'm just like that. And I tried to take, I don't want to disappoint anyone by, like—I don't want to look like a slacker. So, asking my husband to do things that I feel like I should be able to do makes me feel like I'm not pulling my weight. You know what I mean? So, the fact that I'm really struggling to get by at work. I don't want him thinking that I'm like, that I want to stop working because I don't want to help out." Elaine is worried that her need to take naps and manage narcolepsy may be misunderstood as a choice to not spend time and energy on the family and its needs.

Switching back to how affairs are at home, she explained, "They actually sleep really well, there's just so much more to do. Napping during the day can't really happen anymore. Or I guess it could but I got to get stuff done around here, you know." I wonder aloud how does she do it. Then I described how my sisters have an informal rule that I am not a babysitter. Her son had been putting a tent pole in his mouth while walking around, and when he started to whine, she responded, "That's why you don't walk around with them in your mouth." When she returned to this topic she added, "It's hard to manage work and home. Like I'm, like I said before, I feel like I'm sinking sometimes." She walked to the sink to put water into Dale's cup.

Aurora has a similar story because she was homeschooling her children when her sleepiness started to become more obvious. As she explained, "during the day, during story time, or whenever, I could not stay awake. That was the biggest thing with the kids. We had jokes and what not." Once she was diagnosed with narcolepsy she developed cataplexy, but the medicine and treatment didn't seem to work. As she explained: "But at the time, my husband at the time, ex-husband, he, 'You just need to get more sleep.' He didn't get it. 'You're just wearing yourself out. You need to know when to shut down.' He didn't get it." Later Aurora explained that his inability to understand narcolepsy was "the straw that broke the camel's back," because, "in his mind, even if I wanted to fight, I'm not going to fight anymore. I'm just going to use narcolepsy as an excuse and shut down. That was happening because I was so stressed out." Aurora also regrets not being able to do more with her children because of the tiredness that came along with narcolepsy. Narcolepsy, for Aurora and Elaine, means possibly being misunderstood in fundamental ways while also creating a sense of guilt for having limits that impacted how much time they could spend supporting the family.

Home Bittersweet Home

Elaine found fulfillment in the roles and responsibilities of being a wife and mother, and there are indications that being at home created a sense of control and belonging. Meanwhile, home also is a place where her family's misunderstanding about narcolepsy led to guilt and a lack of support which created additional stress. Repeatedly, she reiterated how she felt like she was "sinking" because she never has enough alertness or time to commute to and from work three times a week. At home, narcolepsy may mean endless obstacles to fulfilling one's role as a mother but it can also mean being able to manipulate the situation to carve out time for a needed nap. Elaine's story also demonstrates how geography plays a significant role in navigating narcolepsy.

One issue that does not vary much from one geographic area to the next is the general expectations of parents. There are people who have lost custody of their children because medications failed to alleviate sleepiness enough to allow them to manage the tasks associated with parenting. It is not hard to imagine how devastating such a ruling might be while also bolstering the stigma of having narcolepsy. In one article that explored the topic of parental fitness and narcolepsy, the authors recommend that supporting the parents with child care would go a long way to address parental fears about losing custody (Barbero et al., 2017). Thankfully Elaine largely had this form of support from her family. Nevertheless, the topic of parenting with narcolepsy or other fatigue inducing conditions is an area where more research is needed.

Arthur Frank (1995), in *The Wounded Storyteller,* introduces a concept that might be useful here. Elaine's story resembles what Frank (1995) calls a chaos narrative because of the overdetermination of narcolepsy in her stories and also because of the lack of narrative sequence. Elaine must deal with a sleepiness that is not yet clearly understood and is not yet sufficiently managed by medications. Like the moment of hearing Elaine's story of falling asleep while working with patients, chaos narratives are hard to hear and can provoke anxiety. Our sharing of each other's stories helps our stories invite others to recognize themselves within it. It also points to how the true chaos narcolepsy may create is "the hole in the telling," because vast stretches of her experience of narcolepsy still exist in subjectivities that lack speech (Frank, 1995, p. 102). While Elaine's story reminds me of Frank's (1995) concept of a chaos narrative, the next chapter centers around a testimony narrative that will further explore the dilemmas inherent to driving with narcolepsy.

Chapter 5

Driving with Narcolepsy

The chimerical experience of excessive daytime sleepiness is unique to conditions like narcolepsy and idiopathic hypersomnia. Therefore, it would be a mistake for a person without such a condition to think that their experience of occasional sleepiness was analogous to being disabled by unexpected episodic sleepiness. Sleepiness, for people who do not have hypersomnia, narcolepsy, or a fatigue-related condition, is often a rare and coy feeling that must be patiently courted for individuals to enter the realm of sleep in a timely manner. Excessive daytime sleepiness, on the other hand, is neither rare nor coy in the lives of most people with narcolepsy. Sleepiness is such a challenge that it is difficult to personify it without relying on overly hyperbolic language. For example, excessive daytime sleepiness is somewhat of a demon, a pirate, a thief, and yet it is also a familiar and constant companion for those who live with narcolepsy. Understanding the experience of driving with narcolepsy relies on also understanding life with overpowering yet evanescent excessive daytime sleepiness. Central to meaningfully engaging with the intersection of narcolepsy and driving is the question of trust. This chapter does not want to betray the trust placed in people with narcolepsy; rather it seeks to create a nuanced account of what driving means to Sable and others with narcolepsy.

Popularized depictions of narcolepsy as falling asleep unexpectedly contributes to the idea that driving for people with narcolepsy is inherently dangerous—even if the person in question does not feel sleepy, is on adequate medication, and takes several precautions to avoid putting themselves and others in danger. Indeed, there is no shortage of driving simulation research and survey research that suggests that people with narcolepsy are dangerous drivers (Philip et al., 2013; Phillips & Sagberg, 2013). Additionally, cataplexy is also a symptom of narcolepsy that can impair driving. Some researchers who know about the soporific force of excessive daytime sleepiness and the unpredictable nature of cataplexy argue that people with narcolepsy should have restrictions placed on them by their doctor or the state (Donjacour et al.,

2010; Mets et al., 2012; Philip et al., 2010). However, as blatant as this argument may appear, the absence of news stories in which people with narcolepsy kill or maim drivers and or pedestrians complicates the idea that people with narcolepsy are more dangerous than other drivers (Fitzsimmons, 2016; Trotter, 2014).[1] The relative lack of accident reports associated with a health condition likely partially has to do with the way undiagnosed narcoleptics will not have that information, and because of how sleepiness and cataplexy may itself stop severe patients from putting themselves and others in danger. While both pictures are plausible—narcoleptics as dangerous drivers or as unable to cause harm—the reality of course is somewhat more complicated. This chapter hopes to show a more nuanced understanding of what narcolepsy means when behind the wheel. In addition to the salient yet shifting meanings of danger, cultural messages about driving also help construct the experience of driving while narcoleptic.

Sleepy driving is not unique to people with narcolepsy. In the 2012 National Sleep Poll 80 percent of professional drivers admit to driving while drowsy when they are not working (National Sleep Foundation, 2012). This happens despite 23 percent of drivers knowing someone who has crashed because they fell asleep at the wheel (National Sleep Foundation, 2017). The likelihood of being involved in an accident is not only a matter of personal choice and chance, but it is also connected to the circadian rhythm. The circadian rhythms of most humans make around 2:00 p.m. and 2:00 a.m. the times when the body is more prone to falling asleep (Dement, 1999).[2] In Stanley Coren's (2014) book, *Sleep Thieves,* he reviews the work of Peretz Lavie, who found that traffic accidents peaked in Israel during the hours in which the low points in sleep wake cycle create stronger urges to sleep. These peaks were between 1:00 a.m. and 4:00 a.m. and between 1:00 p.m. and 4:00 p.m. (Coren, 2014). The morning peak is much more severe even though there are fewer vehicles and therefore less opportunities for accidents.

Driving is a major part of the iconography of the United States (Potenza, 2013).[3] While getting a driver's license is still a major milestone in the lives of youth in the United States, each year fewer are choosing to get a license and this may point to a change in U.S. car culture (Potenza, 2013). While driving represented freedom for previous generations, generation Y-ers see the environmental costs of driving, the danger, and the isolation from others and one's devices all make driving less appealing. Knowledge about cars has often been considered a male province since the first Model T Ford came off the assembly line in 1908, more recently the internet allows all genders access to information about cars (Lezotte, 2015).[4] Driving is a way to express, follow, challenge, or reinvent social identity categories such as race, gender, age, class, and ability (A. Cohen, 2014; Julian, 1998; Lee & Molnar, 2017; Pachana et al., 2016; Associated Press, 2014). Driving also represents the freedom of being able to choose where to go at any moment, and people's emotional connection to driving can be seen in the way cars are similar to pets in that owners may both name and talk to their vehicles (Johnson, 2017).

The road movie is a genre of American films that built upon the adventure genre of American literature. In these films, however, the journey is a form of cultural critique and traveling is a way to explore one's self and the world (Laderman, 2002). Driving is a site of diverse subcultures, a site of protest and activism, a site of leisure, and a site of innovation and development (Bijsterveld et al., 2013; Chaudhry, 2017; Fleetwood, 2017; Loewit-Phillips & Goldbas, 2013; Onion, 2015). These and other cultural, structural, historical, and personal factors are at play in driving despite tendencies to communicate about driving in terms of individual responsibility and individual choice.

Sable is fifty-six years old and has narcolepsy with cataplexy. Sable gave up driving many years ago, therefore to explore the meaning of narcolepsy in the context of driving, Sable's second interview occurred while in the front seat of a car. After introducing Sable through her diagnosis story, this chapter will explore the themes that emerged in my analysis of her second interview. Sable's interview revealed two conflicting meanings of driving: narcolepsy makes driving dangerous, and narcolepsy makes driving necessary. After narrating our discussions, the chapter examines how they shed light on what narcolepsy symptoms mean while also weaving in stories from other interviewees. This chapter concludes by arguing that the meaning of driving is tied to the social resources and the roles people have. These resources can alleviate the risk and danger of driving, while the roles people play or seek to play will continue to influence them to find safe ways to drive.

SABLE'S DIAGNOSIS STORY

I met Sable when I agreed to hang out with Jane, who put the support group on Facebook, as discussed in the appendix. Jane drove me to Sable's condo where inside we sat on a sofa in a smoky dark room facing a large patio window where some light poured into the room. I enjoyed meeting new people, but darkness was my kryptonite, so I resisted leaning back onto the chair where sleepiness might be waiting. I was charmed by Sable's kitten who was shyly exploring the room—staying far away from us but close enough for me to admire her. I had a beautiful cat, and rarely encountered cats or kittens that could compete with mine on that metric. Mango was a petite rescue kitten that looked like a mix between a Siamese and a white and gray American Shorthair. Sable and Nancy shared the history of the support group, which is also detailed in the appendix, and agreed to do interviews with me.

The following week I returned to Sable's place for an interview, and this time I told her about my aversion to darkness. After some deliberation we decided to do her first interview in her gated patio at the umbrella table on a bright cloudless day. Now fifty-six years old, Sable was diagnosed with narcolepsy in her second year of college, in 1978. Sable married Joe a few months before she was diagnosed with multiple sclerosis (MS) in 1990, which came after having lived with narcolepsy with cataplexy for many years. Sable recalled having problems with reading growing up. She tried standing up and sitting up to read but she tended to fall asleep while reading even at a young age. She explained, "I had a terrible time with reading. I knew how to read; I just kept falling asleep." In college, she had one semester where she did really poorly because she wasn't able to stay awake during the final exams. The sleepiness was getting in the way of different aspects of her life, as Sable said, "But the cataplexy is what took me over the edge. I mean, I just—I couldn't walk down the hall. Somebody tells me a joke, I'm down at work or school, anywhere. I could fall flat down on my butt." Her cataplexy developed around the age of twenty-two, when for a year, she would experience muscle weakness, so if there was a chair or something she could simply take a seat. Yet standing up was a strategy to help manage her sleepiness. This progressed to falling to the floor. Laughter was her main cataplexy trigger. She tried several medications to control her cataplexy, and nothing worked for a while until a doctor recommended Prozac. Sable went from having three or four cataplexy attacks a day to having two to three over the course of a year.

Sable's dad vehemently rejected the idea that she had narcolepsy. In an attempt to persuade him that narcolepsy was a real condition, Sable brought home a video of dogs with cataplexy but he persisted in refusing to believe it was a real condition. When she disclosed her narcolepsy, it was often greeted with laughter. She recalled, "They thought I was kidding. It was just, 'Oh, I was just trying to get a good laugh out of all of them.' 'No, no, no. This is for real. This is a real illness and a real thing.'" Such reactions did not discourage her from talking about narcolepsy. Like with her father, she persisted. In another conversation, she shared with me that Joe occasionally tries to encourage her to talk about it less. While in college she was in a sorority, but after being diagnosed, Sable said they also were not able to regard narcolepsy as a real thing. Which is why she decided to leave the sorority.

Sable met Nancy, around the age of nineteen or twenty while at a sleep convention in downtown Columbus. As she described it, "We all went out somewhere to get something to eat or drink after this lecture or something. And Nancy went and somehow or another, we just started talking. And she was a local bird like me, and she had the same thing I did. And she was such a sweetheart, a nice person. And I've been in touch with her ever since that day." Nancy and Sable ran the Columbus support group when Jane came along much later and was able to put the group on Facebook where people who are newly diagnosed can find the group. Sable believed, "I needed it most at first. I needed to accept it and understand it."

Sable's diagnosis story features familiar aspects of previous diagnosis stories like the hesitant family member and her struggles around staying awake for driving and working. Sable's story differs from previous narratives because of how her symptoms impacted her education and her prolonged struggle to find medication to help treat her cataplexy. After being fired from a federal government position for her sleepiness, her mother worked with her to find a lawyer to represent Sable and was eventually awarded disability retirement payments. After going months without an income, Sable was able to buy a condo when she was twenty-two; we met in this same condo many times. For some time, Sable was a wheelchair user because, as she put it, her leg "refused to bend." When she was interviewed, she used a walker to get around.

THE LIFE THREATENING AND THE LIFE SUSTAINING MEANING OF DRIVING

One of the early patterns gleaned from my interviews while still in the field was the realization that many people with narcolepsy had car crashes. It makes sense for the personal vehicle to emerge as a major site where the meaning of narcolepsy can be examined. One day while on I-70 heading to meet Nancy for an interview, there was a semi hanging off a bridge with the trailer pointing into the air. To capture this memorable sight, I pulled out my phone and took pictures as I rolled by. People tend to do a lot of unsafe acts behind the wheel, narcoleptic or not. The risk is obvious upon reflection, although at the time it seemed like a reasonable idea. Hindsight often tends to offer better alternatives. Hindsight is a major character in this chapter, always offering value after the fact.

Many interviewees were asked about conducting interviews in their car as one of the salient locations that appeared in their diagnosis stories. They regarded this suggestion in various ways—sometimes silently, sometimes recognizing the logic of it, and other times I rescinded the suggestion forthwith, recognizing how their obligations and commitments make being honest about driving difficult. Sable's reflections on driving come from the perspective of someone who has given up driving, and therefore may serve as a proxy for people, like myself, who are still driving and napping behind the wheel. Her story of driving is an opportunity to examine the practice through the eyes of someone who clung to driving fiercely but eventually decided to give up driving because of her narcolepsy and her MS.

Sable's understanding of the dangerous choices to drive before her cataplexy was under control or while vulnerable to sleepiness seems to be largely shaped by the value placed on her sense of independence and on the life-sustaining meaning of driving to manage narcolepsy. In our interview, Sable wrestled with these contradictory meanings of narcolepsy in relation to driving.

Sable's second interview touched on several ways in which driving was dangerous. She began the interview by clearly denouncing the idea of driving with narcolepsy and then went on to describe the many accidents she had before abandoning the road. Sable's stories about driving reflect on the paradox of driving as a person with narcolepsy, which holds that it is both life threatening while also being a considerable source of independence and agency. She also talked about the various ways she guarded herself against car accidents by having strategies to promote alertness and keep sleep at bay.

The Dangerous Narcoleptic Driver

Once I found her condo with the help of Google maps, I stared at the unfamiliar door wondering if I had the right place or not before leaving my car. Parts of the condo complex seem familiar while others, like the door I should knock on, were harder to recall. Sable greeted me at the door and, once inside, I was excited to see Mango again, but I was less charmed by the little white dog who yapped persistently and wanted to put his paws on me. I greeted her husband before we headed to my car to talk about her memories of driving and the reasons she gave it up. Using her walker, she walked to my car and got into the passenger's side of the car. After getting in the driver's seat, I realized that I should be in the other seat. Rather than making an issue of it, we started to chat about the support group while I fidgeted with my phone to turn on the recorder. My Corolla is silver with a light gray interior and black carpet. It is one of the larger makes because it was made in 2010 during a time when many car makers were increasing the size of all car classes. Since it was a hot summer day, I started the ignition to put the air conditioning on.

After chatting about the support group and not being able to be involved in it anymore, Sable said, "but anyway, about driving . . . I had just little accidents here and there."

I followed her lead and replied, "So tell me about that."

Once while exiting a major freeway, she explained, "I was awake enough somehow to get off that exit and then I faded out again I guess. I rear-ended this person, and they rear-ended somebody, and then they rear-ended somebody. Oh, God, it was a mess. I still didn't give up right after that either."

Going on she claimed, "I remember it was snowing. Windows all the way down and my hands were out the window, I was freezing them off to keep me awake; whatever I could do to stay awake. I made it home, no accidents and all that kind of stuff, but a bunch of things have happened to me when I'm driving and I still didn't want to give it up. If it wasn't for Joe, I still think I would probably be driving." Although she regretted causing accidents and driving for as long as she did, she also wanted to reassure other people with narcolepsy that she would never insist that they cease driving. She stated, "I would never go into a court thing and all that against people with narcolepsy." Later she added, "We all have to give up our driving privileges. I think that we should. In my heart and mind." Then she recognized that this is based on her experience of sleepiness and driving noting, "I feel that there's so many other people that do it every day and never have a problem."

Here she takes three positions on driving with narcolepsy in the interview: driving is something that requires strategies and techniques, driving is a site of a lot of symptom occurrences, and driving is contingent on her social resources and responsibilities.

The prevalence of car crashes in my sample likely reflects two dynamics, (1) the diagnosis that occurred after becoming drivers and (2) the age demographics of the sample (see appendix). These accounts of crashes also reflect what doctors often hear is behind what brings patients to sleep specialists for help (McCall & Watson, 2020). As an enormously heterogeneous condition, there are people with narcolepsy who have never had issues with driving and experience the opposite of being sleepy while behind the wheel. John, for example, has never had an issue with driving and considers himself to be the safest driver he knows. Similarly, Grouse provided a rich account of why he is confident about driving. In comparison to watching television Grouse finds driving to be much more invigorating, observing:

> Well, if you were to compare it to driving. Driving, for me at least, there's more stimuli. There's more kinds of stimuli. You got scenery. You see something over there. You're looking at the cars, "Oh, what model is that?" You got the light, you have the shades the sky and you got the cars zipping by. You got a lot of things bombarding you so that tends to keep me awake. But as soon as I pull in the driveway and come in and sit down on the sofa: I'm gone. That's the tendency.

For Grouse, driving is a type of safe zone where the environment is so stimulating that he is unlikely to be susceptible to sleepiness. As a person who has never or rarely worried about sleepiness while driving, the task of driving affords him capacities that it does not offer Sable and others.

As previously noted, all interviewees were diagnosed after the age when people in their respective generation typically became a driver. It is reasonable to presume that prior to diagnosis, they likely approached their vehicles with the same attitudes most people have around driving while sleepy—utterly unaware of the danger of irrepressible sleepiness unique to narcolepsy. Many car crashes or close calls later they are diagnosed with narcolepsy and prescribed medication to make driving and other tasks easier. For many people this suffices; however, others are dissatisfied because there are no standardized criteria to determine if it is safe for a person with narcolepsy to drive or engage in similar tasks (Donjacour et al., 2010). It is important to note that falling asleep while driving could be symptomatic of several conditions. This chapter is primarily relevant to people who are diagnosed and are under the care of a doctor for managing their condition. Safety concerns arise when an individual's symptoms are not adequately managed (Falvo, 2009), and as discussed previously, it can take years to find the correct medicine and dosage while attaining the medicine remains subject to the discretion of health insurance companies if the patient has health insurance. During this period of finding the underlying condition and appropriate medication, it may mean driving amid varying levels of sleepiness, which calls for having strategies for managing this danger.

Strategies for Managing Danger

Like the discomfort of Sable's sticking her hands into the frigid winter air, there are several strategies for when narcoleptics sense that sleepiness has joined them on their journey. As someone from the deep south, the idea of making yourself cold to stay awake was novel but ultimately dependent on geography and season. I returned to the topic and asked, "When you were driving, how would you try to stay awake? You told me some of the things like keeping your hand out the window even though it's really cold. What are some of the other things?"

She told me, "Radio, songs, whatever. If I had a tape player or whatever, some kind of music."

To clarify I asked, "You would just like put it on, or put it loud, or what?"

"I'd put it on medium loud. Nothing blaring blaring, but just so it could keep my mind activated so it wouldn't go to sleep hopefully. If I had a song going on in my mind. Things like that, I guess."

"Anything else?"

She added, "I can't really think of anything else. I always made sure I had something to drink with me. I figured if nothing else, usually water I could just throw it on my face if I had to, you know what I mean? I remember getting out and putting snow on my head before." African American women tend to develop aversions to putting water near their hair, so this idea of splashing water on my face never seemed like a real option. Wearing makeup regularly would also make the strategy less appealing. After hearing about it as a solution to sleepiness, I began to wonder if it worked.

Out of curiosity I asked, "When did you start doing that?"

Sable answered, "Oh, way back," using her hands for emphasis before continuing, "I don't even know if I was diagnosed with narcolepsy yet. Probably was . . . I must have been twenty-two to twenty-six maybe, somewhere like that."

I asked for a demonstration, and she showed me how she would put water on the tips of her fingers and then flick it onto her face by opening her hand while the palm faced her. If this didn't work, she would simply pour water on the top of her head. I then offered my strategies for staying awake—not leaning back on the seat, singing a song; I even tried calling someone once. On long trips, I would be sure to bring sunglasses because if I needed to nap in a parking lot, the sunglasses might hide my sleep from onlookers.

Moving on to another topic I posed this question, "Were there any kind of thoughts or worries or concerns or anxieties?"

She confided, "Oh, definitely. Always, there would be. 'I feel good,' but I never knew because sleep would hit me somewhere between here and my destination. Usually my destinations were within a half hour's time at the most, but I always just kind of said a prayer to myself and to the Lord and said, 'Help me get there safely.' Most of the time I did, but not all the time."

Once diagnosed, Sable approached driving aware of how narcolepsy placed limitations to how she could safely drive. Like the strategies that Sable mentioned, many people I have interacted with online and in person discussed naps as a strategy for managing unpredictable changes in alertness that may occur while driving. Nancy has a habit of taking a nap before approaching the task of driving to the grocery store. This is how Nancy chooses to manage sleepiness around driving while not placing limits on her ability to drive. Like Sable, Nancy also is retired so she can take three to four naps a day—an option that people who are employed or in school may not have.

Aurora, on the other hand, has her cataplexy under control, but if driving and she started to sense some sleepiness, then, "I have to pull over." She elaborated by adding, "I'm really good at sensing, knowing my limitations. If I need to pull over, if I need to stop, I'm going to because I did have a car accident once." Aurora explained that the accident happened because she was distracted for a second or fell asleep for a second, and before she knew it the morning traffic turned into a three- or four-car pile-up because she missed when the car in front of her started to stop for a stoplight. She learned from the accident, and told me that "Now when I see it, I don't even try. It's like, 'Okay, you're starting to have issues, shut it down.' Don't even . . . 'Maybe I could press through,' is not a friend." Aurora learned the hard way that even if she thinks she feels awake, mornings are not a good time to drive. These days she usually has her son drive in the morning.

Considering their vulnerability to falling asleep while driving, choosing not to go to an event is another way that people with narcolepsy adjust their driving choices. Penny talked about having to turn down invitations to go places because of the issue of driving. For the book club she was a part of, she succeeded in volunteering to host meetings, which meant she did not have to risk driving back and forth. However, when someone on the other side of town hosts them, she would worry and weigh not going up against the possibility of getting into yet another accident.

Dangerous Sleepiness

Wanting to know how sleepiness affects Sable I asked, "What would that, 'Sleep would hit me,' mean? What do you mean by that?"

She admitted, "I just couldn't keep my eyes open any longer. Of course, you can't drive with your eyes closed."

I wondered, "How would that feel? Would you have a feeling, like a heads up, that you knew something was changing, or would it just change?" In other words, did she get warnings about sleepiness or would she immediately fall asleep without the prelude of sleepiness?

Sable stated, "A little bit of both," adding, "but I think mostly that it would just change. It went both ways sometimes, but I know there were a lot of times where I would just go off the road and lay down and sleep in my car or whatever. Joe was working at a computer store down at the Easton Shopping Center. I don't know if you know where that is; but anyway, there's a shopping center down here and there's a computer store, and he was fixing computers and doing computer stuff and all that for his job. We had one car and I was just in during the day toward when he was getting off. I went down to pick him up and for some reason I got real sleepy and I just parked somewhere in Easton Shopping Center's parking lot, just laid down and fell asleep in the car." She gestured that she had a car with a bench front seat that didn't have a console dividing the driver's side and the passenger's side, so she was able to lay down in the front of her car. She would nap in her car a couple times a month, "not every day."

As I considered her description, I realized that this unfolded in a world without ubiquitous cell phones and digital watches. These naps struck me as different from the ones I took even in doing my commutes to and from Columbus but upon further reflection, perhaps her naps are more like mine although it is uncomfortable to acknowledge this.

She revealed further, "I just would wake up when I'd wake up. Usually, I'd always wake up within two hours, it seems like, from my bladder if for no other reason. I'd just kind of rely on that for the most part."

Another way that Sable tried to minimize the danger of driving is by avoiding certain driving conditions. She recounted, "I was trying not to get on the freeway a lot of times, but if I could avoid it, I just thought I would be safer at a slower speed. If I was going to have an accident, I'd rather have it at a slower speed with less chance of me getting hurt, of course, or anyone else. Like I said, I was always running late for work because I hated it so much, I guess, but I'd be racing down that freeway. At the time, I was driving a '62 car, and it was a badass car." Sable continued to use the fact that she had not received a ticket for all the speeding she did, ultimately attributing it to the old car.

I wondered, "So did you ever get a ticket, or did you ever feel like you'd get one? Because when you got in these car accidents, you got a ticket, or did you?"

She admitted, "Oh yeah."

I inquired, "Yeah, so what was that experience like? Did you tell the cops what happened?"

She explained how she got into a car accident while exiting I-270 to get on Morse Road. In her first interview, she described the accident this way, "I rear-ended these people so hard, and they rear-ended somebody, and they rear-ended somebody. And we're talking—these cars are all like Mercedes, Jaguars, these expensive Aston Martin whatever vehicles. And I just felt terrible." This multicar pile-up is an instance that will come up again later in the chapter. Similarly, Sable's answer to the question posed is also addressed later.

After she gave up driving, Sable was still haunted by the accident she caused decades ago and takes full responsibility for it. It is somewhat of an open wound. Since medicine does not eliminate all narcolepsy symptoms, people with narcolepsy are often left to wrestle with the aftermath of accidents on their own (Bayon et al., 2009).[5] As Aurora puts it, after she was diagnosed, "There wasn't any support. The doctor I went to at the time [said], 'You have narcolepsy, here are the pills, bye. Hope you stay awake.' That was it." The support group helped Aurora, myself, and others recognize how not seeing or having access to a specialist who knows about narcolepsy can be dangerous. The preponderance of accounts about doctors who treated participants the way Aurora described suggests that perhaps medical professionals may be morally culpable in an indirect way for accidents patients get into after diagnosis. This is not an argument about fiduciary responsibility, rather it is an instance where perhaps bioethicists and psychologists could explore what it means for a person like Sable to take responsibility or otherwise assuage lingering feelings about a long-ago accident. Medicine is intimately involved in this interaction between place and bodies. Furthermore, doctors, insurance companies, law enforcement, pharmaceutical products, transportation infrastructure, and social support networks are all a part of the complicated interaction between people with narcolepsy and their cars.

For Sable and Aurora, narcolepsy means placing your life and safety in the hands of doctors that may know little to nothing about narcolepsy, and it is here, behind the wheel of a car, where that trust is tested and may be found to be wanting. Sleepiness is not the only aspect of narcolepsy that can make an unwelcomed appearance while behind the wheel, Sable has also experienced cataplexy while driving.

Dangerous Cataplexy

Dealing with narcolepsy on their own does not necessarily mean that they are alone, as I learned when I asked, "Did you ever drive with people, like drive people around?"

She uttered, "Mm-hm (affirmative), yeah."

Surprised, I inquired, "And people who knew you had narcolepsy? Or how did they regard or talk about [it.] How did you talk about your falling asleep in the car with them?" My family and some friends rarely had me do the driving if we were going someplace together—except if they needed a break on a long trip; even this was a risk they rarely took.

Sable assured me, "I would just say, 'I'm sick. I got to take a nap,' whatever, but I do remember one time I was driving and I had cataplexy."

"This was before you were diagnosed?"

She continued, "No, this is after. There's a park here in town called Snowville, and I was over there by the park, because I love the outdoors, and I saw some deer and I got just tickled by that for some reason. That threw me into this cataplectic attack, before I was on medications that worked for that. The doctor tried me on so many different medicines. He goes, 'I'm out of choices now. There's nothing else to try.' Nothing worked, not a thing. He was the one that came up with the Prozac, saying it resembles a class of drug they use in Europe for cataplexy, and it works."

Returning to her story, I queried, "What happened with the cataplexy? How long did that last and what happened?"

She replied, "I would always fall."

To redirect her back to the specific account I interjected, "Well, for this particular [story]—the deer. You saw the deer and then you lost the complete muscle control, or just you felt it go and come back, or what happened?"

She reported, "No, I felt it go, and the girl I was with, she knew about all this stuff. I just said, 'Cataple-xy,' and I was able to point at the steering wheel. I got the car to slow down and stop but I couldn't steer it anymore. She grabbed the wheel and between the two of us we were able to get the car off to the side of the road and all that. That was probably one of the only times I heard what a cataplexy was actually driving, and that scared me a lot." In other words, she is indicating that she sensed it coming on and had time to tell her friend.

Shocked, I concurred, "Yeah, that is pretty scary." We talked further about how she was diagnosed with narcolepsy before she started to experience cataplexy.

I asked, "So, when the doctors learned about the cataplexy, did they ever tell you about not driving or suggest that that might not be safe, or did anybody talk to you about driving with cataplexy?"

She confessed, "Yeah, even with the narcolepsy. Both, yeah. They almost took my driving privileges away one time and I fought it like a dodo. You know, 'Oh, I still want to be Miss Sufficient and go get 'em, this that and the other; nobody's going to hold me back.' I'm glad I finally have come to the understanding that it's not safe, not only for me, but God forbid I would hurt somebody else." Despite the remorse she feels, she also admits that her MS and the support of her husband were a big part of giving up driving, adding, "If it were an emergency, I'm sure I would drive, like if Joe ever got sick and we needed a hospital or something, you know. I can still drive, especially now that I have the use of my left leg. Because my left leg was just . . . It was like I didn't even have a leg for so long because of the MS."

People like Sable have no shortage of disturbing memories behind the wheel to make the appeal of not driving apparent. Yet while the probability of experiencing EDS, cataplexy, sleep paralysis, or automatic behavior can be studied using statistics, the lived meaning of this potentiality exists in the way it occupies our memories and stories. For Sable, it seemed she did not regard the story of cataplexy with the same level of regret and danger as the sleepiness.

Sable's story also reveals that communication is central to dealing with the experience and aftermath of driving while experiencing narcolepsy symptoms. Recall the story of automatic behavior in chapter 2 where my sister pressured me to drive late at night. In both my account of experiencing automatic behavior behind the wheel and Sable's story of experiencing cataplexy behind the wheel, a friend or family member was involved in addressing the situation. In an ideal world, everyone has friends and family members who will take the wheel allowing those with narcolepsy to avoid the dangers of driving all together. Instead, patients often have piecemeal support and guidance for dealing with what might be the most dangerous aspect of living with narcolepsy. Effective patient and family education about narcolepsy may help ensure that the people closest to those with narcolepsy are likely to encourage safe choices.

The Isolated Narcoleptic

Why did Sable continue to drive after experiencing cataplexy and sleepiness while driving? Was she being a "dodo," as she claimed or was something else going on? Perhaps examining what she accomplished through driving will provide insight into her root motivations at the time. As a person who was awarded disability retirement before the age of thirty, Sable did not need transportation to go to and from work every day. In addition to the themes about how narcolepsy made driving dangerous, Sable's interview included themes about how driving was a source of freedom in a life that was curtailed by narcolepsy and eventually MS.

As discussed in her diagnosis story, being diagnosed with narcolepsy meant leaving potential sources of connection and support in the form of a sorority that did not take narcolepsy seriously. Sable was not the only person who sought to move beyond the isolation that narcolepsy can impose. Jane's invitations to talk and hang out and my willingness to accept them both reflect how life with a dearth of energy can lead to a somewhat isolated life. By far, the most socially isolated person in this project was also the one whose profession most resembled my own, Grouse. A librarian at a Columbus area university, Grouse was reticent about talking to his family about his narcolepsy, and when asked if he had someone he could call on during a medical emergency, he mentioned that he could ask people at the university before admitting that, as he put it, "I'm extremely socially isolated." As I discussed in chapter 4, when all the sparse energy and alertness a narcoleptic has goes to work, it can leave barely any energy for anything else. This contributes to a sense of isolation that driving may help alleviate. The themes about the life-sustaining meaning of driving cluster around what Sable was able to do as a person who drove, her resistance to giving up driving, and the impact of accidents on her attitude towards driving.

Driving to Support and to Be Supported

Early in our interview, amidst the talk of crashes and regret, I asked why Sable kept driving. She explained briefly, "Because I loved it. I liked being self-sufficient. I was always a strong person and I never relied on anybody else. I was a self-maker, self-sufficient." She continued, "Now I do feel like I am relying on somebody. He doesn't mind it. It doesn't seem like it." Towards the end of our interview, I asked, "How would your life have been different if you gave up driving at a much younger age? . . . Let's say if you gave up driving that year after you had the cataplexy attack behind the wheel, how would your life have been different? What do you think would be different?" This is a rewording of a question I asked everyone in the second interview.

However, instead of asking what life would be like if she never returned to driving, I had to come up with another way to find out what would be missing if it was not a part of her life.

It took a few attempts to rephrase the question before Sable had a clear sense of what I was asking. She mused, "Wow. It would be completely different, completely different, I think. Something just dropped out of my head. I don't know what I was about to talk about. Hit me one more time with the question." This used to happen to me too. Only when I see it as text do I fully appreciate her turn of phrase, "something just dropped out of my head" because it reflects how these memory snafus feel.

After I repeated the question, she corrected me, "Well that wasn't an accident, I think, because like I said, the girl knew."

I jumped in and clarified, "I just had to pick, arbitrarily, a time period, so that you can think about the role driving had in your life and how things might be different if you weren't the driver."

Sable revealed, "Well, if I wasn't a driver I wouldn't have been able to go to as many places and [do as many] things as I would go to if I were driving. I would have missed out on some things, probably, so to speak." This was true in one sense; however I told her how I recently spent time with Jane, who had been getting around without a personal vehicle for some time. Jane was dealing with a car that did not work, and despite the lack of transportation, she managed to keep herself extremely busy. I clarified, "So if you could get around, if you put that aside, how else would it be different?"

She started back in, "I wouldn't have been . . . I'm just trying to think. I probably wouldn't have gotten the narcolepsy support groups together."

In confirmation, I said, "Okay."

Continuing, she stated, "I never would have met Nancy. I would just be confined to my home, for the most part, I think, at that point in time of my life." In other words, if she gave up driving at an earlier point, as she said, I would not have met her because the support group that Nancy and Sable ran eventually became the one I came to join.

While this type of speculation lacks the type of descriptive function more pragmatic questions provide, it did allow me to witness how she dealt with a challenge. Driving, as it turns out, is a major tool she has used to help cope with narcolepsy, and that realization poses a significant dilemma for people with narcolepsy. My own travels to and from Columbus for my doctor's appointments, research interviews, and participation in the support group are all similarly confounding. This is because driving is clearly a means to enhancing my capacity to understand and manage narcolepsy while also multiplying the opportunities where the consequences of sleepiness may become even more dangerous.

Sable's narrative and discussion of giving up driving include several intimate relationships—her husband, the coworker, Nancy, and her friend that took the wheel during a cataplexy attack. While driving and sleep are often discussed as if people were disconnected from relationships that facilitate, accompany, and/or impinge on these activities, relationships are also central to developing safe and healthy habits around driving and sleeping. Sable's companionship—in the form of her husband—supported her eventual decision to give up driving while her need for friendship and belonging is offered as one of the main reasons she resisted the idea of giving up her driving privileges for as long as she did.

Continuing to interrogate Sable's imagination, I posed a question about what narcolepsy would mean if the issue of driving was not a part of living with it. I was somewhat surprised to hear that the dilemmas of driving with narcolepsy was central to her understanding of how this medical condition places limits on people. This unanticipated recognition likely reflects my position as a person who came to know about narcolepsy before learning to drive, and my own experiences of growing up, going to college and to graduate school where long drives and long commutes were often easily avoided.

Hearing Sable return to her conviction that people with narcolepsy should stop driving, I asked her to consider, "If let's say five years from now most people with narcolepsy avoid driving, either because of legal reasons or because of other reasons, how would your understanding of narcolepsy change in that context? If it wasn't a thing."

She interrupted and asked, "If people were made to give up driving?"

I clarified, "Well, if that just wasn't an aspect of narcolepsy because it was easier. I don't know, let's say there could be a number of reasons why people end up not driving. But if that wasn't an aspect of narcolepsy, how would you think of it? What would you think of narcolepsy then?"

To this, Sable declared, "It wouldn't be near as bad. That's one of the big, big things is my driving with the narcolepsy, I felt." She looked at me to see if I knew what she meant before she continued, "Every time I drove, I knew it was a little dangerous, probably, because I don't know when I'm going to fall asleep. If I can fall asleep standing up, it just happens. I can't control it. I don't know if all narcoleptics are to that degree or not."

Sable seems to downplay the role of medication in treating narcolepsy and making the task of driving a safer proposition. Nevertheless, her assessment of narcolepsy seems to possess admirable simplicity. Yet, its simplicity does not diminish the condition's widespread effects on other aspects of quality of life. Rather than taking Sable's statement about driving literally, it feels more appropriate to regard her statement as a hybrid of literal and metaphorical understandings of narcolepsy. As a metaphor, not driving represents how narcolepsy circumscribes the lives of those who live with it. It also reflects the prospects for people who have severe cases and people whose symptoms are uncontrolled by medication. Even as such, it communicates the limits narcolepsy creates and makes a compelling need for support and understanding seem as modest as an offer to take someone to the store.

Anything to Keep a Driver's License

Returning now to Sable's memories of driving with narcolepsy, her love of driving and her commitment to driving is best illustrated in her story of what happened after the first car crash she detailed. In response to my question about what she did after the pile-up when cops arrived on the scene, Sable recounted, "I would usually make up some other story. Like the one I was telling you: I was getting off the exit ramp of 270 to get to Morse Road, and I just was fooling with my stereo I think or something. My eyes were off the road for a second and that's how I ended up rear-ending this person."

Considering this I said, "So you did say that to hide the narcolepsy or hide falling asleep? Because, you know, a lot of people fall asleep. They may not always tell the cop, but they are either undiagnosed or they had avoided sleep for one reason or another." Since many people's ability to know if they are asleep or awake may be impaired when they are on the cusp of sleep and wakefulness, these self-reports and fibs should not be taken too seriously (Schutz et al., 2013).[6]

More to the point, Sable's previous admission about her willingness to lie to keep her license reveals how dramatic her current position on the topic is from the stance she once took. Her changed stance demonstrates how malleable such convictions can be as time unfolds. Almost as if she could somehow offset how a younger Sable was willing to court various risks for the sake of maintaining her driving privileges. Eventually, Sable started to carpool to work with a coworker, and her husband would also contribute to her having more choices around driving. As previously mentioned, as her MS worsened, driving also became less tenable, but once she regained movement in her legs, she did not seek to return to driving. Perhaps it was the way her life forced her to abandon driving that showed her how to live in Columbus without driving.

A couple of my participants brought up the question that is asked when renewing or receiving a driver's license in Ohio. They ask if you have a condition that causes periods of unconsciousness as a way to target epilepsy (Epilepsy Foundation, n.d.; Kramer, 2009). Cameron said that when she was diagnosed this was one of the first issues she thought about. She feared losing her driver's license and worried that she cannot tell people about her narcolepsy. Narcolepsy is distinct from epilepsy because states may require people to prove they are seizure-free or that medication controls them before being given a permit to drive. And there are reports that this state imposed precaution is unwarranted because people with epilepsy have a crash rate that is half the rate of nonepileptic drivers (Epilepsy Foundation, n.d.). While Cameron's fear of losing her driving privileges may never come to pass, Sable's stories may make anyone with or without narcolepsy wonder what they themselves would be willing to do to keep their driving privileges.

Both Grouse and Sable have told me about being awakened by officers or troopers for napping on the side of the road. Napping in a parked car is one of the ways that sleeping behind the wheel for people with narcolepsy might seem like a safe way to avoid driving while sleepy. This issue of napping in the car is dangerous in another capacity. "Sleeping in a vehicle" is shorthand for a type of homelessness, and many cities have laws against sleeping in vehicles (Bruder, 2017; A. Cohen, 2014; Associated Press, 2014). Similarly, people who seem to be asleep in cars is a fixture of books that cover the opioid crisis although these supine bodies usually have overdosed (Macy, 2018; Temple, 2015). Associations with being unhoused and illicit drug use makes sleeping in a car, even for a short moment, subject to hasty judgments about who belongs and might not belong. People with different identities may have different distinct advantages or disadvantages when an officer approaches such a sleeping driver.

The Ends of Sleepy Driving

As discussed earlier and in chapter 2, my family and friends played a big role in managing the risks of driving in my teens and early twenties. My family's willingness to do the long drives is not unlike the coworker who Sable was able to carpool with and her loving husband who is glad to do the driving. Future studies on how people with disabilities handle personal transportation uncertainties should explore the roles and interplay of relationships and resources. In her second interview, Sable began by denouncing this choice to keep driving, and towards the end of the conversation she reflected on the vital role driving played in coping with narcolepsy.

Greater understanding of narcolepsy may lead to greater access to social resources like carpooling, family and friends who will offer rides, and virtual options for attendance, thereby providing more social involvement options for people who are at a higher risk of falling asleep behind the wheel. Perhaps designers and engineers who are developing driverless cars should consider the needs of people with narcolepsy and similar conditions.

Sable did not rely on driving to sustain employment unlike most of the people in my study. This makes her story and her choice to not drive unique from those who rely on commutes or live alone. Penny, for example, found that she was falling asleep while driving to trainings in the morning but felt, "I have to get there. I didn't have another option; you don't get sick days from your clinical practicum. You go, or you don't graduate." This was prior to her diagnosis and she managed the twenty-minute commute because upon falling asleep the rumble strips on the side of the road would wake her up at least once a week.

Some of Sable's stories around driving with narcolepsy take place in a world prior to when the seat belt violations became subject to primary enforcement, meaning police officers could pull over cars and issue tickets. Whereas it became illegal to manufacture a car without a seat belt in the 1960s in the United States, attitudes around seat belts did not change until the 1980s and 1990s when people could get a ticket for not wearing one (Insurance Institute for Highway Safety, 2017). Attitudes around the risk of driving drunk have also changed dramatically over the last few decades aided by the way laws were enforced (Loewit-Phillips & Goldbas, 2013). One of the major goals of Arianna Huffington's *Sleep Revolution*, which refers to her book and her efforts to change attitudes about sleep, includes the goal of making driving while drowsy as stigmatized as driving while drunk (Huffington, 2016).[7] This is a noble goal in spirit, yet this might also result in stigmatizing people like Penny and Elaine who are already stigmatized. Instead of punitive processes, it might be more prudent to advocate for a world where each person has a surplus of eager and willing drivers in the form of coworkers, family members, friends, neighbors, public transit systems, taxis, and Uber-like options for potentially sleepy drivers and for everyone else. Until then, communicating about narcolepsy may continue to result in undesirable isolation instead of fostering relationships with a measure of altruism and empathy.

Since this research was originally conducted, sleep researchers and doctors have published a number of studies that examine the intersection of medication, narcolepsy, and driving (McCall & Watson, 2020; Sagaspe et al., 2019; van der Sluiszen et al., 2021). This has resulted in improved guidelines for doctors and patients to address the question of driving with narcolepsy. Nevertheless, the meaning of narcoleptic symptoms, in the car and beyond, is intimately tied to the resources people have and the roles a person is expected to fulfill. Life with narcolepsy is a patchwork of decisions even in this site where the consequences of sleepiness might run the highest. After my interviews with Sable, she showed me a colorful collage she made with the earlier support group. It featured the word *what?* in slime green Halloween-shaped letters followed by an orange *narcolepsy* all surrounded by many *z*'s and other words that were also cut from magazines and newspapers. Like this fear-infused collage, the decisions around driving are pieced together based on what is available, and in the end, such a patchwork still looks somewhat daunting. The next chapter takes a decidedly more positive approach to exploring the connection between narcolepsy and place.

NOTES

1. Using the NewsSource database, which accesses forty national and international news papers and over four hundred regional news papers I was only able to find Trotter's (2014) piece that reports on a woman who is a nuisance to residents because she has often been found napping on the side of the road in her car. Only one other news story about narcoleptics crashing vehicles is Fitzsimmons's (2016) article on a person who caused a train crash and was later diagnosed with narcolepsy. These were the only two that did more than "suspect" narcolepsy and even those stories were rare.

2. Dement (1999) notes that people incorrectly assume that the afternoon lull is because of lunch when, "In reality, people are feeling their accumulated sleep debt. . . . In many cultures, people cope with this early-afternoon dip by retiring immediately after lunch for an afternoon nap" (p. 81).

3. In Potenza's (2013) magazine article he shows that in 1983 73 percent of youth between the ages of sixteen and nineteen received a driver's license and in 2011 50.9 percent of youth between the ages of sixteen and nineteen are getting a driver's license.

4. Her essay argues that the internet offers a way for women to learn more about cars and car culture to become more informed consumers, engaged drivers, and better negotiators in male-dominated domains like car sales.

5. Their study found that, "medical treatment does not seem to be completely efficient, and physicians should pay more attention to the education, work, life and social environment of their patients" (Bayon et al., 2009, p. 421). They also argue that in hypersomnia conditions like narcolepsy, sleepiness is far more handicapping than cataplexy although few studies examine this.

6. People who are asleep or transitioning between sleep and wakefulness frequently misreport the state they were in when awoken and asked. People with sleep disorders have an even lower rate of correctly perceiving and reporting their state.

7. Huffington (2016) criticizes the tendency to applaud sleep deprivation as a badge of honor in the workplace when, "the effects of sleeplessness are largely the same as those being drunk" (p. 31). She goes on to say that it is endangering ourselves and others. Her book notably has only two pages devoted to the topic of sleep disorders.

Chapter 6

Active with Narcolepsy

In inviting participants to bring me to a place they wanted to share with me I somewhat forfeited the ability to neatly control the themes of each chapter while also gaining a valued perspective on living with narcolepsy. Accordingly, this chapter is a departure from the pattern of briefly introducing a location as a cultural space that holds many meanings before sharing a diagnosis story followed by an exploration of what a particular space means for the participant with narcolepsy. Rather than bringing me to a place where they struggled with narcolepsy, all the Black participants selected a place where they felt a degree of freedom from or triumphed over narcolepsy. John talked to me at a skate park, Aurora and I visited her church, and Cynthia invited me to her dance studio. Rather than focusing on how one type of space is about being physically active and the other is more about a spiritual community, I was able to identify a shared perspective these spaces offered. These selections may have been in keeping with African American communication styles that infuse expressions with positivity and emotional vitality such as the themes of transcendence found in both gospel music and Black art (Hecht et al., 2003). In selecting these spaces, they were seizing an opportunity to share memories that contained a positive glint in their journey with narcolepsy. Cynthia's voice breathes many lessons of grit and resilience into a book that seeks to reflect multiple perspectives on narcolepsy.

This chapter recounts my time with Cynthia, first at her place of work, then at a ballet studio, before ending with reflections on seeing her perform with the dance company. Her story builds on the insights gleaned in earlier chapters about how narcolepsy impacts life at home and at work while also highlighting what it is like to have narcolepsy while in a community and space devoted to being physically active. For Cynthia, who is forty-two and unmarried, dancing is a place where she is free from most of the ways sleepiness limits her. Then I explore how Cynthia's background and commitment to dancing and her sense of belonging to a dance community socially construct the meaning of her narcolepsy in the context of dancing. The chapter concludes by exploring other relationships to being physically active with narcolepsy before reflecting on how these stories shed light on life with narcolepsy.

CYNTHIA'S DIAGNOSIS STORY

During the meeting described in chapter 3, where I met most of the interviewees in this project, one woman arrived much later than the rest of the latecomers like myself. When she had a chance to speak, Cynthia explained to the group how she was determined to make it to the meeting. About a month after initially meeting, I sent her a text message to schedule a meeting with her. She suggested that we meet at her office, and after giving me the address, she texted, "And I suppose I should mention that I work at a funeral home. Please let me know if you think that being there will feel in any way uncomfortable or disturbing for you." Instead, I was mildly amused by this message because I found her concern for my comfort charming.

I replied, "Thanks for the heads up. Yes, I will be okay," before adding, "That was funny." To explain what I thought was funny I texted, "I look forward to hearing about the more memorable responses to that disclosure."

I was the one running late to our meeting this time, thanks to navigating Columbus rush hour with a GPS app I had begun to distrust. I pulled up to the funeral home where she works and spotted a woman waving to me. I tried the door only to discover that it was locked. I was unsure about the person walking towards the deeply tinted glass doors to let me in. Then I saw her hazel eyes and was reassured that this was Cynthia. She had lost a lot of weight since I met her. Later, after our interview, when she brought me back to the glass doors, she stepped outside and I saw hints of blue in her eyes. Delighted, I asked, "Do your eyes change color?" Smiling, she told me about how they sometimes change with the seasons, weather, and/or the lighting.

She was with clients, members of a Black family who came to see the body or for a viewing—which I presumed was in the nearby room. They were in the process of expressing their appreciation for her work, saying how good a job the funeral home did. I stood near and tried to mirror Cynthia because I was unsure how I should act in this unexpected scene. Cynthia's relaxed smile and serious eyes reassured me that I was not out of place. She was wearing a dark dress with a pearl collar that huggedher neck. Unsure about what was happening, I began to think about how the meaning of this moment was so intense for the mourners, who were strangers to me; and yet it likely meant something entirely different for Cynthia, as who worked at this funeral home, and yet still something different to me. As I stood beside Cynthia, a woman shook Cynthia's hand and told me how good a job Cynthia was doing.

I offered a subtle nod in agreement. When she finished gently corralling the last of the mourners, Cynthia showed me to her office where I began to set up for the interview while she finished her work. This is when I started to marvel at her performance. I suspected that the right attitude and an appropriate mix of patience and urgency was needed when hosting family members and loved ones. In any job, there is an emotional repertoire one must be able to express and endure, and I had difficulty imagining the repertoire she must routinely master.

The interview started when I said, "Alright, now tell me about your diagnosis story."

I sat at a table that was a hybrid between a conference table and a desk. On one end of the table was Cynthia's desk with a desktop computer. This table was likely where she would talk with family members about funeral arrangements. Sitting on the other side of desk, she told me, "Okay—so about roughly fifteen years ago—early 2000s—I really don't remember how I came to go to a sleep doctor, but I was basically diagnosed with narcolepsy." She went on and added, "At that point the doctor kind of explained to me what that meant, and I was told at that time that the only medicine that was available to treat it was Provigil. So that's what I was prescribed. I took the Provigil for maybe a couple of weeks, and I just really had really bad reactions to it." Cynthia has narcolepsy without cataplexy and suspects that she has had it since she was a young child.

As someone who recently discovered that a year of mysterious pain was a side effect of my medication's interaction with caffeine, I was especially curious about her side effects. I probed, "Okay—do you remember what they were?"

She added, "It just really made me feel jittery and almost—looking back on it now I probably was experiencing anxiety." Then she explained how her doctor was incredibly unhelpful, "He was just basically like 'It is what it is and there is no cure for it. Take this medicine or don't take it.'" Hence, she stopped taking Provigil and tried to deal with narcolepsy without medicine. Two years ago, she started to experience different symptoms. She explained, "I started having other symptoms that I didn't even associate with narcolepsy. I was having the really, really bad memory loss, insomnia so I was thinking like: If I have narcolepsy how could I be having insomnia?" She changed sleep doctors. Her new doctor diagnosed her with sleep apnea and narcolepsy and later started her on a CPAP machine for sleep apnea. She went back to the first doctor to see if they were able to help. The therapist she saw for depression recommended finding a support group which led to her discovering the support group on Facebook.

Describing her first meeting, she related, "So, the first time—I don't know if it was the first time I went or the second time I went—well, the first time

I went I think I left like really excited because I was hearing other people talk and tell their stories, and I was like, okay—I'm not crazy. And then the second time I went I was a little bit more vocal about my own situation, and I was like in tears and just breaking down crying the whole time. And so going to that meeting—a lot of the people there had had my sleep doctor, the sleep doctor I'd had before and they were like, 'Get away from him. He's bad news.'" Cynthia listened and found another doctor. The group also was especially enthusiastic about sodium oxybate (Xyrem)—which she had never heard of. Eventually she asked to be prescribed Xyrem. On Xyrem she started to see major improvements in issues with brain fog and concentration, but as a person with high blood pressure she also started to experience a lot of dizziness. She concluded her account by saying, "So, I have had definitely two visits with this new doctor and I'm going to see him again in July. But basically, I'm just still trying to manage it the best I can and not really doing a good job at it. That's about it."

In response I asked, "So, why do you think you're not doing a good job?"

She explained, "Because the whole morning thing." Cynthia, like many people with narcolepsy, has trouble transitioning from sleep to wakefulness in the morning. Since her dad is her boss, she has been able to remain employed, but getting up and getting to places in the morning has been a major issue for her. She pointed out, "Like today I didn't have one so I just had to be here at 9:00 a.m. I got here at noon." She paused and added, "So that's really my biggest obstacle is trying to pull myself up and out of bed and get moving in the morning. The loss of time, even here working; before I know it something that should have taken me maybe twenty or thirty minutes to do, three hours has gone by and I'm still doing the same thing." This in an example of how excessive daytime sleepiness often creeps in and stealthily takes little pieces of life in the form of tardiness, poor memory, poor concentration, and poor performance.

She went on to tell me about the headaches she was having with Armodafinil (Nuvigil). I offered, "Okay, yeah—there are side effects and that's specifically the main one. Some of the times I can nap off some of my headaches." Before moving on to other questions, I want to make sure I understand her story, so I said, "This is what I'm hearing; so you were diagnosed a long time ago, but there has not been a lot of treatment, and you haven't found the right treatment, and your relationship with doctors and medicine has not proven to be as beneficial as you were hoping it to be. You're still hanging in there—does that sound about right?"

Cynthia's replied, "Yeah—that's pretty much it."

Later in the interview, she told me how the funeral business is a family business and her father is the second generation of family owners. In college, she studied electrical engineering but she has been working in the family business since finishing school. He hopes to pass the business to Cynthia but, as she put it, "I just don't feel that I'm ready to take it on. And it's mainly because of me like being tired and being—like I can't stay on top of all the responsibilities and remembering everything that has to be done." This has gotten worse since her mother passed away thirteen years ago since she took on all her mother's possessions but has not been able to get her house in order because everything is so overwhelming. She continued, "I tend to focus more on work, my personal life, and my home life, and all of that suffers because I can't focus on all of these things and get all of these things done." Cynthia was able to go around the corner to her parents' house if she needs a nap during a workday. While Cynthia's dad recognizes her need for naps to manage her condition, Cynthia's stepmother does not and tends to wake her up from naps to do tasks around the house. Both her work and her home responsibilities leave Cynthia feeling drained and depleted, which is part of the reason dancing is tremendously meaningful.

I asked, "So, tell me about the dancing. Do you see narcolepsy appear when you are in that kind of an environment or is that a narcolepsy-free zone?"

She told me that, "ninety-nine percent of the time it's a narcolepsy-free zone. Well, I take that back. It used to always be a narcolepsy-free zone." To talk more about her narcolepsy-free zone we agreed to meet at the studio where she danced.

CONTROLLING THE BODY AND LOSING THE BODY

Before continuing with Cynthia's story, I would like to introduce the theoretical lens I am using to understand Cynthia's experience. Berger and Luckmann's *The Social Construction of Reality* approaches the idea of reality as a question of how subjective experiences become objective facts (Berger & Luckmann, 1990). In other words, how does the subjective experience of narcolepsy—a questioned and complex condition that disfigures a hidden and often underacknowledged physiological process of sleep and wakefulness—become real for both non-narcoleptics and narcoleptics? In other words, social construction allows us to assess how narcolepsy is rendered external through interactions and therefore able to be incorporated into how people see narcolepsy despite all the ways it remains hidden.

Life with a condition like narcolepsy means struggles, and needs are often silenced by virtue of being surrounded by people who often fundamentally misunderstand the nature of the condition and its symptoms. My earlier chapters discussed the many ways in which people with narcolepsy must figure out how to deal with excessive daytime sleepiness at work, at home, and behind the wheel. While Sable found help and support for her need for transportation and found understanding in the support group she started with Nancy, the quest for support and acceptance is unending for most of my interviewees.

The absence of people who understand and empathize with the experience of living with narcolepsy also became a familiar fixture in my life. It eventually became an accepted aspect of everyday life such that when I was first offered an empathetic comment about life with narcolepsy from someone who did not have it, I was moved to tears. Twenty years of talking about narcolepsy taught me that it tended to be regarded as some sort of mental illness, an excuse for being lazy, a weird illness, or as a taboo topic for conversation—it was rarely regarded by others as a disability, a limiting health condition, and a source of constant frustration and curiosity. Eventually people who spend time with a person like me may come to learn such truths about narcolepsy. But meanwhile the available information about the condition often fails to communicate what narcolepsy meant in everyday life, and in turn these interactions socially construct the condition as hidden and suspect. These experiences compound to work to socially construct the meaning of narcolepsy in everyday life. Since socially constructed realities are fragile by nature and vulnerable to breaches (Mehan, 2010), when somebody acknowledged that they could see what narcolepsy means in my everyday life, it breached my sense of reality, and I was, for a moment, not alone in my understanding of my life. In a sense, this also happens for Cynthia at her dance company; when she nearly falls she is embraced by people who were able to truly see narcolepsy and the limits it puts on her life and hopes.

Narcolepsy is not a contested illness because it did not endure the public scrutiny that post-traumatic stress disorder, multiple chemical sensitivity, and chronic fatigue syndrome faced. The etiology, physiopathology, treatment, and effects of narcolepsy have been thoroughly studied and were never in dispute within modern medical discourses (Swoboda, 2006).[1] Rather, narcolepsy is a rare condition and therefore similar to contested illnesses in the way in which people with narcolepsy struggle to explain their symptoms to doctors and others (Swoboda, 2006).[2] Another point of similarity is in the way people with narcolepsy may be treated as if their condition has a moral or psychological basis (Japp & Japp, 2005).[3] People with rare conditions frequently do not have their everyday needs met, and this impacts their participation in areas of everyday life and much of this is because of contextual barrier factors (Jaeger et al., 2015). Consequently, the goal of my ethnographic descriptions of conversations and narratives of people with narcolepsy is to provide rich descriptions of the nature of these barriers and to create evocative accounts of how they are dealt with. Accordingly, this chapter provides accounts in a context where side effects were experienced, but instead of finding barriers and resistance, Cynthia found support in dealing with the consequences of nearly falling in ballet class.

In Cynthia's story and in the stories of my other participants, the dialectic of controlling the body and losing the body emerged. Nowhere is this dialectic clearer than in the realm of being committed to being physically active. Cynthia's lifelong involvement with dance requires assiduous control over her body, and yet narcolepsy creates the need for this type of leisure while also impinging on it. When her dance instructor sees Cynthia's struggle for control over her body, the silent struggle of living with narcolepsy is revealed. Finally, someone sees Cynthia as a person who is wrestling with side effects, and a rare moment of empathy occurs in part because she is in a community of people who also are struggling to master their bodies. After describing the themes that emerged during my analysis of our interview discourse, this chapter will discuss my experience of attending the production of the ballet company and explore how the story of *The Wonderful Wizard of Oz* sheds light on the social construction of narcolepsy.

Controlling the Body

I arrived to the dance studio at 6:26 p.m.; finally on time. Cynthia met me in the lobby and I asked for a tour. The building smelled of new maple wood doors and new industrial carpet. Large windows were cut into the studio walls so we could see through where people in one studio are stretching and chatting before a class. Most people there are White women between the ages of twenty-five and fifty-something, but there are a few people who fall outside of that demographic in terms of race, age, and gender. I was impressed with the stylish exposed air conditioning ducts that allow for the high ceiling. She told me about *The Wonderful Wizard of Oz* ballet that they are putting together. As she showed me where the woman's bathroom was, I failed to register it as a possible dressing and changing room.

The building was wheelchair accessible with a long gentle ramp leading us to the back door. We headed out to find a quiet place to chat.

I mentioned the drops of moisture I felt while Cynthia and I set up three folding chairs between the cars near a handicap parking spot and the loading zone. We faced two residential garages and two attached houses facing the nearby residential streets, and the dance studio was to our backs. We chatted for several minutes before I turned to the topic at hand, "Why do you think it's a narcolepsy-free zone?"

Looking up towards the sky and the trees shading us, she first said "hh-mmm," before tentatively starting, "I think it's a narcolepsy-free zone again because it's my way to, even though I'm physically moving, it's still a form of relaxation for me. It's my way to decompress from the day, to burn off energy and stress." Using her hand to get something out of her eye, she continued, "I can tell when I've been more sleep deprived than usual, I can tell it in my dancing and it actually works in the alternate way. If I haven't come to dance, like if I get really busy at work and I can't get away to come to classes and I go more than a week or so without dancing, I can tell in my mood," gesturing to the building.

For clarity, I asked, "Tell me, what do you mean?"

Sitting with her legs crossed with her phone perched on her leg, she explained, "If I'm busy at work. Usually most of my classes, they're here in the evening, but if there's for some reason that I have to work late or something and I miss class."

Then I probed, "Okay, so you say during the day at work, your mood feels different. You feel like what? What is it like?" Cynthia nodded at me and hummed in agreement.

Cynthia offered, "It's just kinda," lifting her hands and shaking them in to communicate tension, "more, I don't know. More tense."

Dancing helps manage her stress and, like most exercise, it brings several benefits. As I continued to talk about her relationship to dancing, I learned that she has been dancing since she was three years old. While many people in her family are creative, since she never pursued dance professionally, some people in her life have wondered why she would spend a considerable amount of time on it.

This reminded me to ask her about the downside of this place, "So, is there anything you don't like about this place or that worries you or creates any kind of anxiety?"

She started, "There's nothing about this place per se . . . "

Then I added, "Or dancing."

She explained, "Yeah. That worries me or gives me anxiety. I do get frustrated with myself when I don't execute things the way I should," putting emphasis on the word *should*.

Nudging her forward I said, "Mm-hhmm, like, give me an example."

Tentatively she started, "Just certain things, like certain movements that I think—I'm hard on myself because of the fact that I've been dancing for so long, and I feel like I should be a professional at it or something," then she chuckled at herself.

Recognizing humor in talking about being self-conscious, I added, "Or that your body is—are you comparing yourself? Because this, talking about how long you did it, are you comparing yourself to the past?" This was something I saw a lot of participants doing: comparing themselves to the pre-narcolepsy person.

Cynthia admitted, "Yes. Yes, and I try not to do that. I think I did it a lot more. I think I've gotten a lot better about not doing it, but yes. I would really,

really compare myself to the eighteen-year-old me. . . ." Laughing, she went on, "versus the forty-two-year-old me, and then that's another part where the narcolepsy creeps in is because I can't—she might say, 'Here do this,' and I can't pick it up as fast and retain the combination."

This is where my two dance classes in college should start to come in handy. To show that I know what a "combination" means, I interjected, "Like remember the four things that you're supposed to do."

Today the dance instructor was teaching Cynthia the solo for her role as the Lion in *The Wonderful Wizard of Oz*. They recorded it to allow Cynthia to spend more time mastering it while at home since she is prone to memory lapses. This issue of getting more time to learn prompted me to ask, "But, the classroom environment, how is that different from other ways of learning?"

This line of questioning leads Cynthia to paint a vivid picture of dancing as a form of physical activity that emphasizes nuanced control over the body for a sustained amount of time. The picture she painted is later contrasted with her story of losing control of her body because of medication side effects.

Answering my question about learning, she said, "I don't know, I think it's probably—and again, I think this varies. I'm sorry."

I tried to reassure her, "It's fine."

She added, "This varies with the culture of the studio. This studio is relatively relaxed compared to some other ballet studios where they're doing classical instruction, they're very strict, they're very rigid."

Curious, I inquired, "Yeah, tell me about it; what does that mean?"

"If you're taking classical ballet classes, a lot of times there might be a dress code. We were just talking about that because we wanted to."

Jumping in, I interjected, "Oh, like wearing the same outfit or you have to buy their outfit and wear it."

"Yeah like leotard tights." Then she added, "The studio that I grew up in as a child, everybody had to wear black leotard, pink tights, pink ballet shoes. Hair pulled back in a bun, no what my teacher called 'junk clothes.' So, no t-shirts, no legwarmers, nothing extra. Just leotard and tights and ballet shoes. Here, she's not like that. You can basically wear whatever you want. There's different degrees just depending on the culture of the studio where you are. Then the same thing with the discipline as far as the studio I grew up in, you stood a certain way. If you were in the middle of receiving instruction, there was a certain way you had to stand or if you had to sit down, there was a certain way you had to sit."

"It's just T-stand?" I recalled something from my five-year-old dance classes.

"Yeah like we had to stand in B-plus." My face showed my ignorance, consequently Cynthia stood up and showed me the B-plus position—which was more elaborate than the simple fourth position or first position. Her hands were out to her sides a foot or so from the waist; her weight was on her right foot while her left big toe touched the ground behind her modeling the tense yet elegant pose. She added, "like this—the whole time."

"Oh, wow," I remarked.

She continued, "We couldn't just be like—if you're standing there on the side of the classroom and she, the teacher is showing you something, you were standing like this." Now returning to her seat she continued, "If you had to sit down, you had to sit Indian style, with your legs crossed and very straight up and down and your hands resting on your knees and that's always. Just like with the military, you're always standing at attention or at ease; we were always standing at attention." It was different at this studio where, as she said, "here it's very much more laid back." Returning, at first, to the description of more rigid dance environments, she recalled, "You couldn't talk without being recognized by the instructor. Well here, at least for the adults, she's dealing with grown women so she very rarely—now if there gets to be too much side conversation in class, she'll be like, 'Okay you guys need to be quiet.'"

I chimed in, "Yeah, like I can't hear myself."

She confided, "But other than that, people speak out and say things. It's funny because you can always tell the people who grew up with classes with training versus people who are new to dance because they're more like, 'hey!' Just talking."

To show I follow, I added, "Because they don't have the frame of reference that this [studio] is liberal, we can't push this. Just because we can talk doesn't mean." I continued to think about the picture of dancing as the meticulous control of the body and shared some of my thoughts, "Yeah, I see. That is so interesting. I can't help but think about that, because the picture you're painting, a really great picture of an environment where your body is expected to be always in relationship to your will and always under your control, right? . . . Because you don't have always that kind of rigid control over any given moment." I am referring to the clumsiness and accident-prone nature of excessive daytime sleepiness, but Cynthia's inability to control her body came not from narcolepsy, but from the medicine she was given to treat narcolepsy.

Cynthia has a complicated relationship with dancing. This is a place where she can escape the double-bind of unending responsibilities at work where she feels always on-call and the unfulfilling and overwhelming home life. While brain fog may affect her dancing, sleepiness is not something that happens in the dance studio—which is why it can be called a narcolepsy-free zone. This interest in exercising control over her body conflicts with the way narcolepsy undermines it through hampering her memory and through troubling medication side effects.

Losing the Body

In Cynthia's first interview she told me about the dizziness she experienced when she was on sodium oxybate (Xyrem), which is taken at night to help people with narcolepsy get deep sleep. All drugs come with the risk of side effects, and this drug is no different. Referencing her side effects, I asked about narcolepsy while not wanting to say the word, "in terms of your unique issue, how did you get to—were you worried about it making an appearance here or how did that unfold?"

At this she smiled, uncrossed her legs, and proceeded to tell me that it came down to needing to give up dancing because of Xyrem although the medication helped with her memory, which helped with dancing. She explained, "When I started on Xyrem, that had a big effect on my dancing." Looking at the trees and the garage, she tiptoed into the story, "It was kind of weird or emotional. I had gone to a class I couldn't, I couldn't" she was momentarily distracted by a passing car as she searched for the word, "My equilibrium was all off. So anytime I bent over or got ready to do turns or anything," she bent forward in her seat to demonstrate and twisted her hands, "I was just losing my balance and about to black out. I got very frustrated and I walked out of class early and was just upset and crying so after class."

To clarify the timeline, I asked, "And you stayed gone for the rest of class?"

She continued, "Yeah, stayed out for the rest of the class. I was just in my car crying in the parking lot, and she walked past my car and saw me sitting in the car. That's when she was like, 'What's going on with you?' Because she had never seen that out of me before. Then I told her about it and basically for me it was scary because dance is something that I've done since I was three years old." She told Sarah, her dance instructor, that she had a sleep disorder and that she was on a new medication and that she needed to choose between this medicine and dancing. Cynthia explained that she was crying and frustrated with being forced to pick between the two.

Sarah's response to her was, "Don't stress about it. Don't worry about it." And she told Cynthia that she would do research to see if there is a way to find alternative moves for people with equilibrium issues. Cynthia was on Xyrem for only a short time when she was put on a different sleep medication, and her issues with dizziness dissipated.

This is a striking story for several reasons. This situates the meaning of medication and treatment—often regarded as generally good and worthwhile—in a context where I can see how this medication affected her life. It created a major dilemma—Cynthia felt as if she was being asked to sacrifice a lifelong passion to get treatment for a lifelong illness. Her visible struggle and her willingness to tell her dance instructor about her narcolepsy and the side effects she was dealing with constitute a rare story about narcolepsy disclosure because instead of being met with confusion, misunderstanding, derision, or apathy, Sarah responded to the crisis with empathy and support for Cynthia.

These types of interactions around narcolepsy and treatment socially construct an understanding of narcolepsy that is connected to a community of people who are there to support and help each other. The role of family members, friends, coworkers, and educators remains the same when dealing with someone with narcolepsy. Their reaction to and response to narcolepsy helps socially construct the meaning of the condition. For Cynthia, the meaning of her condition is tied to how it is a source of tension and disaffirmation with her family and her career prospects. However, in the company of dancers, her memory problems and the dizziness become issues comparable to other nonprofessional dancers Cynthia's age, and as such, they can be similarly addressed and accommodated. The ballet company works with a few people who are much older than Cynthia, and that means fostering an environment with a certain degree of flexibility to enable people with different levels of ability an opportunity to dance together.

Active with Narcolepsy

Being active with narcolepsy was central to several other interviews with overlapping characteristics. John is a very busy man with narcolepsy and sleep apnea. He is self-employed and married with most of his children already out of the house. An African American who went to graduate school, he is fairly unguarded in telling me that he has difficulty relating to the experiences of the mostly White middle-class women who make up most of the Columbus support group. During our first interview, John's diagnosis story started with him breaking his ankle twice while skateboarding, which alerted his doctor to the possibility that his bone density was low which is associated with sleep apnea in men (Liguori et al., 2017; Sforza et al., 2017).[4] His sleep test revealed narcolepsy and sleep apnea and he was prescribed treatments for both. He turned to his phone during our interview and described how, "Because when I'm sleepy—so even right now, you see me on my phone and I'm gonna play a game and eventually I won't be able to contain it. I already see that. So, I do things to keep me awake." When we met at a skate park, he told me about how he thinks about his adventures in the favelas of Brazil, where he met his wife, as being like the skateboarding—they were all ways of self-medicating to become more awake and more alert. Unlike many of the people I interviewed in Columbus, John has not talked to his family about his sleep disorders because he suspects that they will not understand it. There are many types of activities that John sought to help him keep excessive sleepiness at bay.

Levi, Aurora, and Sable are also participants that enjoyed being active. Levi enjoyed spending warm windy days on the lake wind surfing. Aurora tended to do physically active jobs to keep her on the move, like newspaper delivery, but was now trying a more sedentary job that was engaging in other ways. Although Sable has significant limitations because of her MS, she still loves to dance. During our first interview, Sable told me a story that may illustrate why some people with narcolepsy may be reticent about being active—tactics that may ultimately fail to continuously keep sleep at bay. She started by explaining how attending rock-n-roll concerts are a rare but special treat because of the expensive tickets. At a concert by someone like Stevie Ray Vaughan, a blues guitarist, where, in her words, it was "loud, loud. People are screaming and yelling. And good ole Sable, fall right asleep . . . I could fall asleep anywhere doing anything at any time." While some people have safe zones, like dancing, skating, or running, there are others like Sable who are vulnerable to sleep everywhere.

THE WONDERFUL WIZARD OF OZ AND THE SOCIAL CONSTRUCTION OF ABILITY

The day I saw Cynthia's Facebook post about *The Wonderful Wizard of Oz* ballet I added it on my calendar and told her that I would be there. It was November and months have passed since I last saw her. The day of the event was the day after I took my first dosage of Xyrem. In conversations with other narcoleptics I heard that the first few days on Xyrem could be bad. Accordingly, I was unsure about committing to the three hours of driving attending would require. I messaged Cynthia letting her know that I would need to play it by ear to ensure I felt alert enough for the drive.

The morning of the ballet, I woke up refreshed for the first time in ages—I had forgotten that sleep could feel restorative. My body was full of surprises. I jogged a little more than three miles on the bike trail that winds through a park and partially wooded area in town. My Apple Watch awarded me with a workout achievement for burning more calories than any previous workout. Halfway through the day I decided that I was going to the ballet; so, I finished up my grading and left a few minutes later than ideal.

I showed up to a mysterious building about five minutes after show time. The building had no signs to reassure me that I was in the right location. I drove around the parking lot in hopes of seeing someone else but only saw parked cars. As I left my car, I spotted two women approaching the doors that had a sign indicating that it was the stage entrance, but where was the real entrance? Together we ventured around the outside of the building until we came across the entrance. While walking, we wondered about the high school band noise blaring from the direction of an apartment complex that bordered the parking lot. After purchasing our tickets, the volunteers ran off to fetch three folding chairs for us to sit in. There was only one printed program between the three of us.

The ballet had begun, Dorothy was dressed like the Dorothy in the Judy Garland movie with a blue and white plaid overall dress atop a white turtleneck. Then a little dog made a cameo when he walked onto the stage where Dorothy picked him up. The audience was delighted—for the rest of the show Toto was a stuffed dog. Dorothy soon became sleepy and went inside the miniature house. The music changed indicating a new scene, and soon women with dark gray sheath dresses and black tights entered using motions that led with their arms as if being pulled and then pulling back. They swirled around the house picking up speed and slowing down to dance in place always with long sweeping gestures. There was an occasional pirouette before they departed and another scene began.

The ballet included a number of scenes that I had trouble placing within the familiar movie. I later realized that the ballet was based on the book more than the movie. I will not narrate the whole ballet, but I wanted to offer a sense of what I saw. Many of the scenes were choreographed as group performances with costumes, music, and themes that parallel the story of *The Wonderful Wizard of Oz*. Then there weresolos; each of Dorothy's friends had a solo, plus the wicked witch and the wizard. Places and things in the book were also dancing proxies in this ballet. The wind, the yellow brick road, the forest, the poisonous poppies, were all embodied in dances and clothed in emblematic costumes. The pale-yellow dresses and Dorothy's silver ballet slippers were drowned out by the harsh stage light, but the effect is clear. It was around the time Dorothy met the Tinman, a man in gray overalls painted silver with a funnel on his head, that I started to see a connection between my project and the ballet. Eventually it donned on me, and I inaudibly said to myself, "My interviewees are like Dorothy." They are both misfits who must navigate various places that are often inhospitable to them. Like Dorothy's need for help and companionship, my interviewees also need, and in some cases, find, help and companionship in navigating the spaces I highlighted in this project.

When it was time for the group of familiar friends to take the stage, I was enraptured in the ballet and the allegory it offered. Cynthia seemed to be one of two women of color in the production. Dorothy, the Tinman, and the Scarecrow were having a picnic when Cynthia appeared as the Lion, in a golden sequins and tulle tutu that matched her golden curls. The Lion started to slowly creep towards the picnic, putting her index finger over her mouth to communicate her intention to surprise the picnickers. She soon befriended them and the stuffed Toto before they mimed having a conversation about what to do next. They danced with the yellow brick road before they all exited the stage leaving Cynthia to perform her solo. One of her roar-like moves was when she picked up her knee tucking her foot under her and put her hands curled into a claw next to her ears. She did her dance solo to a piano cover of "Brave" (originally released by Sara Bareilles and covered by Piano Tribute Players). Even though it was an instrumental, the familiar words about being brave imbued the performance and my viewing with meaning. It reminded me of my hopes for my research and how both my participants and me can, at times, be burdened with uncertainty about whether we should speak up about narcolepsy, and at other times we have benefited from this type of encouragement.

The Lion's dance had a mix of ballet, African, and jazz moves, and was the only familiar cover in the ballet. Her solo was a celebratory dance in gratitude for the forgiveness and friendship she found in three strangers. As I watched, I was also celebrating what I found through this project and through the relationships that may outlast it. As Dorothy, the Tinman, the Scarecrow, and the Lion journeyed on and overcame obstacles like the deadly poppies, the witch, and the wizard, I thought of how important the help of others was in living with the challenges of narcolepsy. The voices of the people who have narcolepsy—their brilliance, love, and courage—are a source of friendship, support, and encouragement for those who are in need of it. Only now, a year after starting the project, could I recognize precisely how much I needed their companionship.

On the drive home I was invigorated by the performance and the insights it provided. I was so enamored by the allegory that I decided to read the original book *The Wonderful Wizard of Oz,* by L. Frank Baum. This is how I discovered that the connection between my project and this American fairy tale were even stronger than I had suspected. Furthermore, I was delighted to eventually learn that *The Wonderful Wizard of Oz* had been interpreted as being about the social construction of disability (Eyler, 2013; Haller, 2004).

The Scarecrow, the Tinman, and the Lion were all told that they were deficient by someone they mistakenly trusted, and as a result they came to view their actions through the prism of this flaw. In the case of the Scarecrow, in the original book he was only two days old when a crow sat on his shoulder and told him, "'If you only had brains in your head you would be as good a man as any of them, and a better man than some of them. Brains are the only things worth having in this world, no matter whether one is a crow or a man'" (Baum, 1900, p. 48). The Scarecrow had recently been abandoned by his creator, which is why he trusted the only creature that came to keep him company, and this outlook shaped his understanding of the world. Later that day when he met Dorothy, he was convinced that his naiveté was because of his brainless state and never came to see it as a feature of youth. Throughout the adventure, the Scarecrow was the first to come up with novel ways to address the issues they encountered, and before the Wizard of Oz left, he told the Scarecrow that he was the wisest and wants him to rule over Oz. Each character's disability is similarly socially constructed in this way, and they are all utterly unable to see how brilliant, loving, and brave they are until the wizard tells them a different story—providing them with a narrative prosthesis (Eyler, 2013).

Some cultural critics, such as Alissa Berger (2012), approach the legacy and the original text *The Wonderful Wizard of Oz* arguing that, "The variations of text and performance which follow Baum's work must therefore be engaged on the merit of their individual forms and cultural contexts rather than as 'copies' of a theoretically ideal 'original'" (p. 34). However, over time the story that was clearly about the social construction of disability inevitably has undergone both subtle and dramatic changes, where it has been transformed into a tale that presents disability in the ways that Baum was critiquing (Haller, 2004). Beth Haller's (2004) review of the Broadway production of *Wicked* is scathing, pointing out that in the Broadway show, "disability equals evil once again, and the 'punishment' for disability is death," because the wheelchair-bound character in *Wicked* was cured by the ruby slippers until she is ultimately crushed by a house (para. 11). While highlighting the social construction of skin difference, the book *Wicked* and the Broadway production *Wicked* unravel Baum's tale of the social construction of disability. Today's era of standardized testing came even despite all the critiques of intelligence testing and the problematic pedagogy of teaching to the test. Therefore, perhaps Baum's original story about the social construction of disability has never been more salient.

When I taught about the social construction of reality, I told my students about the Scarecrow before asking them if they know any Scarecrows—people who are brilliant, beautiful, confident, brave, or caring, but are unable to see their true abilities because someone they trusted judged them incorrectly. I was humbled to hear them recognizing Scarecrow in their friends and family members. The stories I have shared in this book compose a part of the ongoing and unending social construction of disability, and as such, it is important to be clear about the relationships between bodies, the environment, and social construction. The context of being physically active allows narcolepsy to be socially constructed as a disabling based on how such a condition is attached to messages and fears about punishment. Instead of receiving negative messages that constructed her experience of narcolepsy, Cynthia was embraced and accommodated when she was told about the possible ways she could dance despite her side effects and narcolepsy. Like in Baum's book, both the Scarecrow and Cynthia are offered a narrative prosthesis to extend beyond the story that limits them (Eyler, 2013). In other words, the Wizard offers the Scarecrow and all his friends, except for Dorothy, an alternative story to allow them to see the world and their bodies differently. When put beside other participant stories about communicating about narcolepsy, Cynthia's narrative prosthesis offers the rare construction of narcolepsy as something that is worthy of empathy and support.

Being Together with Narcolepsy

As discussed earlier, this chapter is a bit of a departure from prior chapters because Cynthia wanted to talk about her narcolepsy-free zone and because the difficulties she experienced there came from side effects and not narcolepsy symptoms. Side effects are a major part of having a condition that involves taking medicine every day and/or every night which means there are other participants who mentioned the side effects they encountered. Cameron, who was one of the recently diagnosed participants, recalled her reaction when the doctor delivered the news: "I'm not going to be completely normal and that I am going to need medicine for the rest of my life." Like a lot of the other recently diagnosed participants, Cameron also still had the habit of comparing herself to the pre-narcolepsy self while wishing she could do more. Medication is a major asset that helps many people with narcolepsy catch up and keep up with others. The medications and the side effects they bring are a part of everyday life with narcolepsy. Although these medicinal interactions are often kept out of sight and may not even be publicly visible, they are a substantial part of the work that goes into managing a condition like narcolepsy. It is only fair that in a book that amplified sensory details also amplify this regrettably ongoing bodily dimension of life with narcolepsy.

To review, Cynthia was forty-two years old, although she was diagnosed when she was twenty-eight. However she spent many of the earlier years without medication and was unhappy with her medical treatment. She worked at her family's funeral home and was expected to take over as the owner despite her doubts about her capacity. Her family knows about her condition and she can sometimes take naps during the day when needed. The support group has been a big help for Cynthia, who felt enormously alone in her struggle, and encouraged her to ask for Xyrem. This drug came with the side effect of dizziness which made dancing difficult. When Cynthia told the dance instructor about her concerns, she was comforted and found that the instructor was very willing to try to make it work. Cynthia, however, was taken off the medicine and was able to continue preparing for her role as the Lion in the performance of *The Wonderful Wizard of Oz*. The ballet and the original story of *The Wonderful Wizard of Oz* is an allegory for this project and the voices within it. The next and final chapter will reflect on elements of this qualitative journey before forging a pathway forward in both disability research and understandings of everyday life with narcolepsy.

NOTES

1. In her argument, Swoboda (2006) focuses on how the emergence of a new illness is a social process in which illness sufferers are involved in the formation and representation of the illness through interactions with medical professionals and large institutional forces. Narcolepsy is legitimated because its interactions with medical and scientific institutions construct it as a valid and therefore not a contested illness.

2. Participants in the Swoboda (2006) study thought that the lists of symptoms associated with contested conditions were broader than chronic illness conditions which contributed to the difficulty in being viewed as legitimately sick and also made diagnosis difficult. This is somewhat similar to the way people with narcolepsy are often misdiagnosed before receiving the correct diagnosis.

3. A person's moral character is put into question when friends, family members, and medical professionals begin to believe that the symptoms originate in the patient's mind. Questions about authenticity and exaggeration raise challenges to the ontological integrity of the self and, "The resulting dissonance, shame and self-doubt can be extremely debilitating, as suffers ask themselves: 'Do I have the right to consider myself ill? Am I lying or deceiving myself and others? Am I taking advantage of others' generosity and good will'" (Japp & Japp, 2005, p. 112).

4. In this exchange between Liguori et al. (2017) and Sforza et al. (2017) both authors discuss why their studies on bone density in sleep apnea patients have had diverging findings.

Chapter 7

Exchanging Stories of Hidden Disabilities

Writing about my time with fellow narcoleptics while examining how place affected how narcolepsy was experienced called for a unique approach to present both the stories and the collaborations of communicating about narcolepsy. The success of this writing, in part, lies in its capacity to help readers access the sensorial and emotional drama of living with narcolepsy while also animating the medical constructs endemic to the condition. This research also seeks to stretch the field of health communication by exploring narcolepsy in a manner that intends to cultivate compassion for a group of people with no shortage of communication frustrations around silencing conditions like narcolepsy. After continuing to reflect on the larger lessons learned, this chapter will first reflect on the intersection of my Black identity and my hidden disability. Then it will reflect on the stories about narcolepsy in everyday life to address the patterns they presented. This chapter concludes by exploring possibilities for new ways to communicate about narcolepsy and addressing issues that future research on hidden disabilities that center identity and place may consider. Narratives and stories are woven throughout.

Let us begin by recalling a few of the somewhat distressing moments in this book: the moment of waking up at a stop light not recalling the drive, the husband who rejected his wife's narcolepsy diagnosis, the multicar accidents, the discussion of falling asleep while working in a patient's mouth, and the dilemma of needing to pick between medication or dancing. Of course, different readers may select other moments to recall here. Now take a moment to contrast these accounts with the medical description of narcolepsy in chapter 1 which reflects how medical professionals and patients learn about narcolepsy. The distance between the medical description and the more gripping personal moments reflects the original intention to be an interlocutor who by sharing my story of narcolepsy with interviewees could elicit narratives of everyday life with narcolepsy and forge a richer understanding of the potential obstacles people with similar conditions may face. These and other insights have immensely enriched my understanding of this peculiar condition and have deepened my empathy for the challenges that exist for adults who find themselves needing to reconfigure their lives to adjust to life with narcolepsy. Though I was diagnosed as an adolescent, there are undeniable parallels between my experiences and that of my participants. Such mirroring moments in this research journey remind me of the curse of Medusa, who was once beautiful and became hideous as a punishment. More specifically, her reflection was a weapon that was used against her. Hence, as an ancient image, the face of Medusa adorned a wide range of artifacts in Ancient Greece, symbolizing a danger that warned of worse dangers (Glennon, 2017). Each account of falling asleep in inopportune moments is also a symbol that warns of yet more egregious dangers people with narcolepsy may face. The relative isolation that may befall a person with narcolepsy is perhaps a catalyst that can make each risk even more perilous.

Sharing one's own story about narcolepsy with peers and beyond is merely one way to bridge the gulf that can be created by persistently being misunderstood and disbelieved. Despite the plethora of ways people with narcolepsy can connect with others, there are countless challenges that may also get in the way of actively participating in support groups online or in person. The discovery that narcolepsy is an autoimmune condition means that each person with narcolepsy may also face several other health conditions that may compound hardships and can potentially undermine the search for effective treatments (Ohayon, 2013). Since other conditions were beyond the scope of this inquiry, there is no way to know if other health conditions may be impacting the participants. Similarly, this investigation limited consideration of family background, socioeconomic status, and psychological factors that can have a profound impact on how well someone may be able to adjust to life with narcolepsy. Despite these limitations, the narratives and analysis provided a rich and rare glimpse into communication about narcolepsy.

Countless absences due to sleepiness and mental fog seem central to life with narcolepsy and yet there are layers of meaning making that can unfold differently along a myriad of identities and places. The analysis of the interviewees sought to elucidate a set of communication patterns that have limited usefulness in terms of generalizable conclusions that are often found in more quantitative forms of research. Nevertheless, the rich descriptions of life with narcolepsy and the communication dilemmas shared here are inextricably connected to the identities and backgrounds each participant brings to the table. Take for example, a public performance artist whose performance entails lying down in public outdoor locations as a clever way to raise awareness about chronic illnesses (Lambert, 2021). Such performances also likely rely on having a social identity that may comfortably enter and exert control over such public spaces. Hence, the contested issue in respectability politics may similarly shape how people of color comport themselves in heterogeneous and homogeneous spaces. Rather than seeking to establish a clear position on the nature of respectability politics or the extent to which it is influencing participants, it is but one of many lenses that can be deployed to scrutinize the intersection of narcolepsy and race.

BLACK RESPECTABILITY AND HIDDEN DISABILITIES

After finishing a series of history documentaries, my partner and I were looking for something new to watch via a streaming service. Once we selected documentaries, an image filled the screen. It was a woman laying prone for a documentary called *Unrest* (2017). My curiosity was piqued, and thankfully he was also interested in seeing it. As the documentary moved forward a vaguely familiar woman detailed her struggle with chronic fatigue syndrome (CFS). Eventually it became clear that Jennifer Brea was central to creating the documentary, which chiefly featured moments from her life along with scenes of different protests that sought to show both the debilitating toll of CFS and the efforts to impact both medical and political systems in the United States. The main similarity between CFS and narcolepsy is the mysterious lethargy that can befall both groups which creates an opportunity for crip time that may or may not be congruent with institutional structures (Kafer, 2013). Another similarity is in how the conditions can confound attempts to create and perfect meaningful self-representations in the form of books and documentaries. By the end of the documentary, I was confident she was the same woman who I saw in a wheelchair for a TED talk several years ago discussing her struggles with chronic fatigue syndrome. One major difference I discussed with my partner that evening was the utter absence of effective treatments for people with CFS.

The documentary also featured many intimate scenes focused on other people with CFS, which was a powerful example of nothing about us without us, a principle of the disability rights movement and disability studies. While the African American struggle for civil rights was a model for the disability rights movement and its various iterations, there is often a tenuous relationship between being Black and having a disability which can take various forms. Chris Bell (2011), the noted disability scholar, said that, "Too much critical work in African American studies posits the African American body politic in an ableist (read nondisabled) fashion" (p. 3). More recently, Leroy Moore (2020) has noted that the recent influx of books on systemic racism by Black academics since the publication of Michelle Alexander's *New Jim Crow* in 2011 have repeatedly failed to explicitly address the intersection of

Blackness and disability. I furtively searched for an acknowledgment of the compounding impact of ableism in Ibram X. Kendi's (2016, 2019) books, in Heather McGee's (2021) *The Sum of Us*, Keise Laymon's (2018) *Heavy*, and Richard Rothstein's (2017) *The Color of Law* but was ultimately too disillusioned to be disappointed with the authors. Perhaps the people who stand to benefit from the unchallenged and deep-rooted ableism of academia are ill-equipped to address ableism in their writings and research. Initially I sought to address my life and narcolepsy without explicitly addressing race. Existing in academia as a Black disabled woman requires an even larger stockpile of grit and daring that I eventually may attain (Bailey, 2017). This conflict is similar to when Robin Boylorn's (2017) grandmother objected to her research, despite the fictionalization that would protect participants. Instead of it being about how, "it just makes us look so bad," referring to how outsiders would see their family secrets, as in Boylorn's work (2017, p. 16); in writing about my life, I must similarly wrestle with the unintended consequences and unpleasant feelings connected to elucidating some of the secrets of my narcolepsy. Since it is a hidden disability, the option to maintain the elusive benefits to remaining quiet on this front has notable appeal. One major frontier that persists in health communication and disability is the issue of Black respectability politics.

I would like to first detail briefly some of the background and meaning of Black respectability politics before making more explicit connections to the book. Black respectability politics has a long history and is connected to John Henryism because its resemblance to John Henry who is a Black folk hero whose belief that his brute determination and hard work proved that he could do seemingly impossible feats. Henryism has been linked to higher levels of diastolic blood pressure and has been explored in a range of disciplines (James, 1994). For Black women, respectability politics suggests that determination to regulate one's behaviors and emotions can lead to positive outcomes. In one qualitative study of Black women in academia, such attitudes were connected to intensified racial battle fatigue, which means that the efforts to reduce the impact of racism inevitably led to heightened stress that could take many forms (Okello, 2021). In other words, Black respectability politics implies that if a Black person could avoid sleepiness and mistakes they might be rewarded with increased acceptance and increased fatigue all while this person may never be permitted to put away the extra work and extra determination that exists to prove that such people are worthy of the life and love others may take for granted.

My autoethnography of growing up alludes to the politics of respectability in the African American community which tells young Black children and professionals that to be embraced by the Black community and White professional spaces, one must avoid certain associations that may evoke stereotypes like poverty, laziness, or lewdness. By performing Blackness, in a way that uplifts both ideals about Whiteness and Blackness promising young adults should be able to move in both spaces with ease. W.E.B. Du Bois's (1903) concept of the talented tenth is often evoked in discussions of the role Spelman College and Morehouse College play in the advancement of Black leaders in both private and public sectors. Similarly, keeping one's personal "business out of the streets" is central to maintaining face in the Black community and in similar interpersonal contexts as well. Despite the embrace of certain forms of disability, like blindness, in the Black community (Smith, 2019), people with hidden disabilities and illnesses are often encouraged to keep their conditions to themselves until they have a positive success they want to celebrate. This double bind that discourages Black people from publicly disclosing a hidden disability is not a problem that needs to be solved, rather it is a layer of complexity this research sought to explore. Similarly, the Black academic community is often reticent to champion people with disabilities due to their proximity to everything Black respectability politics seeks to avoid. Simply writing about these dynamics and barriers does not dismantle them.

The Black Lives Matter movement undermines Black respectability politics by pointing out how a moment of indiscretion or a mistake, such as wearing a hoodie or going to the wrong house to pick up a sibling, should not result in violent encounters the way they did for Trevon Martin and Ralph Yarl. Black respectability politics suggests that individuals can respond to and change structural racism while Black Lives Matters is a movement that seeks to bring an end to both Black respectability politics and the deadly encounters like the ones mentioned above (Obasogie & Newman, 2016). I seek to join the many voices who have similarly begun to interrogate the usefulness of Black respectability politics.

The social identity of the person with a hidden disability impacts how they navigate their condition and the medical system. I can only conjecture about how my identity may have impacted the relationships I developed and the meetings I attended. My unambiguous Blackness means I am often vulnerable to racism while in the field and in the doctor's office. There is a plethora of research on the nature of how racism is experienced for Black patients that I will not get into here (Grandner et al., 2016; Hoberman, 2012; Kreps, 2006). Rather, I hint at this dimension of my field work to underscore the way identity impacts which stories are told and which stories may be held back. In acknowledging one moment of discomfort, I seek to retain the confidences of my participants while also raising the topic as a worthwhile direction for interpretive and health communication researchers to consider. Both racism and ableism often silence and disorient those whose lives are most shaped by these forces. It took considerable soul searching to bare what was shared in this book and go against deeply engrained habituation of remaining silent about the intersection of race and disability. There are countless other silences that remain undisclosed and yet take up space as both a syncope and testimony. These silences might be explored by community members who are willing to turn to their respective groups as both an insider and outsider—as a researcher and participant, as I did here. This qualitative research surfaced more questions than answers at the intersection of race and disability, which is appropriate because the field of Black disability studies is relatively new (Schalk, 2022). Furthermore, I hope that health communication researchers who examine the intricacies of identity in health contexts may continue to explore how identity-based concepts like Black respectability politics and Black Super Woman syndrome may impact how Black people communicate about disabilities and health. With these hopes in mind, I must also acknowledge that the unique experience that formed my identity means that people who have different identities may inevitably draw contrasts between the dissimilar iterations of Blackness and what I have explored here. I eagerly welcome further explorations of disability and Blackness from the vast range of disciplines and perspectives.

NARCOLEPSY IN PLACE

A faculty member walked beside me from the plane to the airport terminal. As we took in our first glimpses of the Las Vegas terminal, she mentioned, "The airport toned it down—the terminals used to be much brighter and louder." She went on to wonder if the environment changed because the noise made it hard for travelers to hear flight announcements.

"Is that right?" I said while nodding. As I followed her and the other passengers, I tried to envision missing lights. Where would more lights be? As I tried to picture the absences she mentioned, I eventually realized how more lights and loud sounds would likely overstimulate some people on the autism spectrum. Instead of sharing this alternate motivation for changing the look of the terminals, I decided to turn my thoughts to the days ahead. Perhaps this conference trip will be full of surprises.

As it turned out, the hotel where our conference was held was too dark for my liking. In the hotel lobby area, the black ceiling made the space feel bigger while also accentuating the sea of fluorescent lights atop countless gambling machines. This darkness paired with the numerous gambling gardens planted throughout the hotel's corridors echoed the airport's deep gray interior. The dim lighting against the darkness created the impression of a never-ending dusk. Similarly, the dimly lit conference rooms and hallways affected me in ways the architectural designers and conference managers may not have anticipated. Parts of my brain can start to get foggy from merely recalling these dim spaces and my inability to turn the lights on to expel a sleepiness that is typically cued by the darkness night offers.

This aversion to darkness partly reflects repeated events where I could observe this effect. When I worked as a substitute teacher, I was in control of the degree of darkness that would accompany the frequent DVD movie many teachers left for unplanned absences. I dreaded falling victim to sleep while working so I would rarely darken the room if it could be avoided. Nevertheless, this relationship between my narcolepsy and place nurtured a curiosity towards what other patterns may emerge between narcolepsy and place. Early on, I learned that no one was averse to darkness in the exact same way that I was—no one else seemed to mind the dimly lit Strongwater room as a place to meet or Sable's dimly lit condo.

Variance between bodies can be seen in how spaces are navigated and in how the physical world is engaged. Subjective experiences are often unable to make claims about causality, which is the domain of objective language. Alternatively, storytelling can communicate how place and interactions have an effect. In affecting us, place participates in shaping how reality takes form (Stewart, 2007). Stories allow us to communicate about sense-making that recognizes the continuous processes of adjustment and transformation.

Statements about generic places are contingent upon the idiosyncrasies of a person's narcolepsy. In other words, while narcoleptics may be able to sleep nearly everywhere, every narcoleptic cannot sleep simply anywhere. Elaine, for example, avoided watching movies because she was not able to stay awake during them, while others have rarely fallen asleep while watching movies. Place interacts with narcolepsy differently based on the specific way sleepiness manifests for each individual and in conversation with the archive of memories that map on to a particular place.

Similarly, being in a car, at home, at work, or physically active presented the people in my project with different possibilities. As Falvo (2009) points out when discussing the meaning of disability:

> A health condition that results in a disability for one individual may not result in a disability for another individual with the same health condition. Therefore, the degree of disability an individual experiences as a result of a health condition depends on the individual's goals as well as those facilitators and barriers that are present in the physical and social environment. (p. 5)

Many of the barriers that my participants faced emerged from the social environment—the attitudes of coworkers, the others not believing their accounts, the inability to nap, the unavailability of other modes of transportation, and the isolation that often accompanies narcolepsy. Furthermore, the social support and resources a person with narcolepsy has may contribute to or detract from their ability to navigate everyday life. Turning to others with narcolepsy allows for a collaborative process of shaping each other's understanding about a condition. This collaboration is fulfilling and validating personally while contributing to how those who are invested in supporting people with sleep disorders understand its impact. Nevertheless, these conversations alone cannot make time lengthen, secure safe passage for sleepy drivers, or undo any of the countless other ways narcolepsy ceaselessly chips away at what my participants hoped for each day. There are several ways health communication researchers can continue to explore the ways that place influences how individuals understand their symptoms and communicate about their needs. The post-COVID-19 world of telehealth and mobile health creates opportunities for methodological and theoretical innovations on this front.

NARCOLEPSY IN EVERYDAY LIFE

To further explore narcolepsy using the theoretical framework of social constructionism, I will, once again, put my observations and analysis in conversation with Berger and Luckmann's (1990) *The Social Construction of Reality* to examine how meanings emerge in everyday life. The meaning of narcolepsy in everyday life diverges from the medical description of the physiopathology, symptoms, treatment, and tests—which is what narcolepsy means to sleep specialists and doctors. The meaning of something emerges not out of dictionaries and textbooks. Rather, as Berger and Luckmann (1990) observe, meaning is in our understanding of reality and, "Everyday life presents itself as a reality interpreted by men and subjectively meaningful to them as a coherent world" (p. 19). The meaning of the world is subjective and is shaped by how people think about it and act towards it (Berger & Luckmann, 1990). Hence, the meaning of narcolepsy is subjective and is similarly shaped by how people think of it and act regarding it. This book sought to uncover many of the meanings embedded in the lives of individuals in specific places to highlight how the meaning of narcolepsy and its symptoms vary depending on the context, the individual, the severity, the familiarity, and other factors. Despite the utter singularity of each possible meaning of narcolepsy, meanings cluster in important ways, and they cluster around different spheres (Berger & Luckmann, 1990). Therefore, the meaning of narcolepsy will tend to reflect relations and expectations of a specific context and individual.

In these different sectors, according to Berger and Luckmann (1990), there are things that are either familiar, or things that are unfamiliar. Our sense of reality is based on being able to maintain everyday routines. Excessive daytime sleepiness and cataplexy tend to be perceived as problematic in part because they often emerge as unpredictable and therefore may disrupt everyday practices. Even a routine of taking a nap regularly can be perceived as disruptive if it does not fit neatly inside of how a workday should run. Meanwhile, even as a problematic part of a workday, the meaning of narcolepsy is further shaped by how a person with narcolepsy might use different routines which will bring about a different sense of reality. Berger and Luckmann (1990) claim that when someone encounters another person who is no longer in a common world where they have a shared sense of reality, the outsider is perceived as "mad" (p. 24). People with narcolepsy often occupy a spatiotemporal reality that is different from non-narcoleptics; they are in different worlds. Still, people with narcolepsy can invite others to join them in their worlds where sleep and wakefulness are not mutually exclusive (Berger & Luckmann, 1990).[1] Through autoethnographic and performative writing about the everyday life of people with narcolepsy, I sought to immerse readers in the alternative spatiotemporal worlds of people with narcolepsy if only for a moment.

My participants often found themselves in situations where they were a misfit—when their bodies failed and/or did not fit the expectations of a space or activity (Garland-Thomson, 2011). This misfit often comes in the form of diminished alertness or cataplexy. The concept of a misfit is useful because it encourages us to focus on what people do when they find themselves not fitting the expectations of space or time. In occupying a subjugated position, people with narcolepsy may possess subjugated knowledge about their unique embodiment. Consequently, the support group can be understood as a type of community where they can support each other and help each other navigate medicine, work, home, and driving (Garland-Thomson, 2011). A lot of the coping I witnessed, participated in, and received was both effective and adaptive, meaning that, according to Falvo (2009), effective and adaptive coping behavior reduces stress and enhances attainment of a person's fullest potential. Coping can be encouraged by the social environment or it can be discouraged by that social environment (Falvo, 2009). The case study approach to exploring the relationship between narcolepsy and place allowed me to collect intimate narratives that revealed how people with narcolepsy coped with a hidden disability.

There are many ways participants reacted to misfitting in their narratives—they adapted, changed, persevered, or took a nap. For example, when Elaine knew that she needed to take her son to the hospital and knew her sleepiness was not yet under control, she *took a nap* to ensure that she was going to be awake and alert. This is something I was once extremely reticent to do, but I have since begun incorporating naps into my day to better manage sleepiness. When Cynthia found that her dizziness was going to make dancing impossible, at first, she cried and received support, then her medication was *changed*; hence, she could dance again without falling. Cynthia also *changed* her mind about hiding her narcolepsy from her dance instructor. Sable initially *persevered* in driving despite several accidents, but as her body changed and once she could get around without driving, she *changed* her position on driving while narcoleptic. Penny used technology to *adapt* to the needs of teaching all the while *persevering* until her doctors identified the appropriate medication and dosage for her. When I ran into her at the sleep doctor's office, she happily reported, "This is what it is like to be normal!" In my autoethnographic chapter, I described each of these forms of coping: I changed, I adapted, I persevered, and I took both voluntary and involuntary naps. Collectively, meaning across the differences that exist among people with narcolepsy, dealing with narcolepsy in everyday life means continually changing, adapting, persevering, and napping. Using writing that shows rather than tells, this text somewhat performatively enacts this way of being a person with narcolepsy (Denzin, 2003).

While subjective meanings will vary widely, narcolepsy means having a brain that does not organize sleep and wakefulness the same way it is organized by non-narcoleptics. This difference gets marked in various ways and may have consequences in the form of being tardy, being fired, making mistakes, getting into accidents, and experiencing isolation. These types of experiences may construct narcolepsy in negative terms when they occur in the absence of meaningful empathy, understanding, and belonging. Alternatively, as Cynthia's story shows, misfitting can be a site of empathy, understanding, and belonging. Having those types of reactions to the absences that narcolepsy creates facilitates everyday meanings of narcolepsy that lack much of the doom and gloom foreshadowed in diagnostic descriptions of the condition.

The theoretical framework of social constructionism emerged out of the stories, observations, and analysis I performed. Ethnographic research encourages researchers to let the field experiences guide analysis and sense making, and this meant that perhaps additional theoretical language would emerge during the research and writing process (Lindlof & Taylor, 2011). Social constructionism surfaced as key towards the end of the field experiences, but it also provides a way of making sense of the earlier stories and problems the book sought to address. Perhaps medical descriptions of narcoleptic patients as unemployable and uneducable participate in the social construction of narcolepsy as such. Of course, if one believes the impact of discourse and language is less influential than one's immediate relations and embodied reactions, this is not a strong concern. Nevertheless, medical discourse is often easily amplified and legitimized in ways that interpersonal communication is not. This is to say that although I argue that the meaning of narcolepsy is constructed in everyday interactions, the legitimacy of narcolepsy remains inextricably tied to medical descriptions that may unintentionally contribute to the discursive stigmatization and marginalization of people with narcolepsy. The challenge of communicating about narcolepsy is further compounded by the accounts where participants felt like their physician had failed to adequately educate patients, family members, and others about narcolepsy. The American Academy of Sleep Medicine and other organizations can address this concerning pattern with the help of patient advocates, communication researchers, and communication design experts.

OCCASIONING SOCIAL SUPPORT IN SPECIFIC CONTEXTS

To better understand what happened when I fell asleep while talking to an office mate, I needed to be in conversation with people who have narcolepsy and similarly wrestled with alertness. This investigation officially commenced when I found myself in the seat of the other person. There I was, sitting in front of Cameron, my first interviewee, confused about what I saw on her face. Was that sleepiness? Was that anxiety? The hope of telling the story of narcolepsy from multiple perspectives is only partially successful since there is no way for me to undo the lifetime of knowledge I brought into this journey. Being across from a potentially sleepy narcoleptic while in public was jarring in hindsight, but in the moment, a surplus of uncertainty caused me to freeze. Considering having sat in the seat of the spectator who was forced to guess what was unfolding inside my interlocutor's brain yielded questions about this positionality. For starters, what is the most supportive way to be a husband, friend, parent, or coworker in the moment someone unintentionally falls asleep? Which considerations best support them at work, at home, and in other locations where sleep is not expected but it none the less appears? Dyadic research into couples, or parent child pairs, might be an opportunity to examine the choices supportive partners make and their impacts to develop guidelines to help families navigate these unique scenarios.

All participants received an early version of the manuscript to provide feedback and to corroborate my observations. The participants who were highlighted and quoted were each given a copy of their chapter and the entire work to provide me with feedback on what appeared in the manuscript. Several participants acknowledged that they read the manuscript and appreciated this member check process. The support group is currently still on Facebook, and I am the main organizer despite having left Ohio and two attempts at recruiting additional leadership in Columbus to host physical meetings as discussed in the appendix. The initial leader sometimes engages the online group. The wrist bands Jane passed out in the meeting where I met most participants were worn unfailingly for years until they each ultimately broke. While the feelings I felt towards bracelets may have varied from time to time, overall, they personified the sense of belonging that this type of research seeded and nurtured.

This book is a practicum on incompleteness. It may help people deal with the never-ending state of lack that is not limited to the experience of narcolepsy—not knowing enough, not being active enough, not feeling enough. The ability to control a disorder like narcolepsy is what Wolf-Meyer (2012) calls a dual-faced situation. It permits control over the symptoms and offers a sense of self-efficacy, but it also requires "compliance," which is not a simple request (Wolf-Meyer, 2012, p. 11). Maintaining health insurance often requires having a full-time job or another source of income, and if that is in place, compliance also often requires the care and interest of family members who must deal with side effects, doctor visits, and the financial dimensions of treatment (Wolf-Meyer, 2012). Narcolepsy, of course, threatens a person's ability to maintain a source of income, trusted family members, and health care. These are all facts that could be deduced from research on narcolepsy alone. The stories told by my interviewees, and the process of researching, both move beyond accounts of peculiar absences to reveal rich glimpses into how people with narcolepsy operate in intimate relationships.

Through interactions with others, narcolepsy transformed from a source of absence into an interaction situated in a spatiotemporal context. When my participants fail to fit into dominant spatiotemporal rhythms, this is an instance of what Garland-Thomson calls misfitting. As a support group, they were able to turn their shared tendency to misfit into a shared identity (Garland-Thomson, 2011)—members could empathize with not being able to make it to a meeting and, hence, there were several meetings where no one showed up. Like the comparisons that Elaine did that placed the accommodations offered at work beside the ambivalence she encountered at home, being able to miss a support group meeting can be placed beside the inflexible obligations and evaluated accordingly. In many ways, the attendance of the support group also waned, in part, because of all the support communication that unfolded on the Facebook page for the group or in other similar online venues. This format unfortunately does not completely replace the experience of hearing someone put an un-named personal experience into words because spoken language makes subjectivity "more real" to both the audience and the speaker (Berger & Luckmann, 1990, p. 37). There are numerous benefits and drawbacks to the centrality of Facebook in the support group as it may bring to any support group. These reflections on the support group participation ultimately yielded a curiosity about how support groups focused on conditions that may create isolation and involve fatigue, sleepiness, or tiredness may navigate the paradox of organizing around a condition that limits social engagements.

The pattern observed in the participants who poured their alert time into work suggests that the mental health of people with narcolepsy is likely also impacted by the time debt that accrues when unexpected naps and difficulty getting out of bed both steal countless hours day after day. The condition itself incentivizes hyper attunement to oneself in an attempt to control or anticipate sleepiness. Similarly, the presence of comparisons to a pre-narcoleptic life as an adult suggests that there are many opportunities for people with narcolepsy to develop unhealthy patterns of self-talk and self-appraisal. Healthy sleeping habits and medication can go a long way to improve alertness, but these alone are not sufficient to address negative patterns of thought about oneself or about sleepiness that are likely to take root in the lives of people with narcolepsy in one form or another if unabated. Compounding these circumstances, people who take a popular sleep medication must abandon alcohol consumption and potentially imperil the socializing and relaxation that some may deeply crave. While the majority of the participants worked full time, their need for more meaningful social support along with a shared reticence around requesting ADA accommodations, seemed to reflect the newly diagnosed status of spotlighted narratives.

STORIES OF NARCOLEPSY AND COPING WITH NARCOLEPSY

As mentioned previously, prior to this research, the constant presence of discussions about medications among people with narcolepsy initially baffled me. It was not until my relationship with my medication suddenly became more complicated that I understood their information seeking behaviors more personally. Exchanging stories about narcolepsy provided me with language and belonging while also offering pragmatic suggestions about medication, side effects, and doctors. Pharmaceuticals are often key to having a sense of self-efficacy over efforts to manage symptoms and to being able to establish goals that sleepiness might otherwise sabotage. Perhaps the most promising thing I gained from hearing the stories of fellow people with narcolepsy is an enhanced ability to imagine a fulfilling future with narcolepsy.

In her book *Narrative Imagination and Everyday Life*, Molly Andrews (2014) explains how asking people to share narratives means putting oneself in a position where one must suspend disbelief to follow the storyteller's tale. In listening to my participants' stories, I needed to be open to novel possibilities about what narcolepsy may mean in a person's life. The stories highlighted here as case studies are moments where my travel companions succeeded in introducing meanings that were entirely new to what I was previously capable of imagining. Andrews (2014) argues that our freedom relies on our ability not only to see things as they are, but it also depends on our ability to see things as they are not and, therefore, begin to imagine a hoped for reality. Knowing about the support and care Elaine's employers offered her should help others imagine nurturing relationships with employers. Discovering that Penny's husband eventually came to accept and understand her narcolepsy may help others imagine similar transformations in how their family members think about narcolepsy. Moreover, these combined stories of people with narcolepsy should empower sleep professionals to imagine people with narcolepsy as people who are themselves remarkable accomplishments considering the lack of meaningful support many of them recount. People with narcolepsy should be capable of imagining niches of spatiotemporal placements where they are not disabled by constraints of social arrangements or physical affordances. These stories should enhance the world's capacity for imagining people with narcolepsy and similar conditions as productive and valued members of society who may require adjustments to allow for daytime sleep. In short, this book should help readers imagine a world where it is acceptable for people like me and my participants to sleep everywhere.

New Communication Frontiers

One of the early discoveries in my interviews with people who were newly diagnosed with narcolepsy was the way conversations provided an opportunity to put into words profoundly internal experiences of sleepiness. This context of conversation called for creating and hearing new words and new combinations of words to communicate about our bodies in a way that reflected how we made sense of narcolepsy. My participants did not explicitly disregard medical language because it also was used by them. But in using the language of symptoms, there often is some measure of doubt conveyed as to whether it is being deployed correctly. Moreover, as I point out in chapter 1, some of the terms like "excessive daytime sleepiness" and "sleep attack," which are commonly used to define and describe narcolepsy in medical literature, fail to help people with narcolepsy communicate about their subjective experiences in their efforts to educate family members and friends. One of the major roles of language in the social construction of lived experience should be to index subjective meanings (Berger & Luckmann, 1990). When Sable responded to a question by noting that her thoughts "dropped out of her head," her description had a clarity that the term *brain fog* could not accomplish alone. Therefore, perhaps the deployment of terms that are more felicitous to the lived experience of narcolepsy may remind concerned parties about dimensions of narcolepsy that are relevant to fostering relationships of support and encouragement. Discovering new terms to describe symptomology is somewhat beyond the scope of the present study, but this direction can be taken up by health researchers interested in expanding the language at play in sleep medicine. Meanwhile, the heavy lifting the word *sleepiness* does for people who are often stranded in this between sleep and wakefulness suggests a thirst for a richer vocabulary to describe the many layers of subjective experiences that unfold between being asleep and awake. Ineffective language about this condition also likely increases levels of stress for patients.

LOOKING FORWARD TO CONTINUING RESEARCH ON HIDDEN DISABILITIES

The future holds several challenges and opportunities for communication researchers, medical practitioners, and people with chronic illnesses. One hopeful frontier comes in the form of something that already exists in the United Kingdom. Chronic Illness Inclusion is an organization that began in 2021 as the product of a social action research project that Jenny Lyus and Catharine Hale participated in beginning in 2017 (*Our History*, 2018). They essentially take a research-based approach to learning about what life is like for people with energy-limiting chronic illness (ELCI) and they propose policy changes to legislators based on their research. In the United States there are a range of organizations that advocate for different categories of health conditions already, so perhaps another organization would have less of an impact than one would hope. Conversely, since many health policy and patient organizations in the United States often depend on funding that comes from large companies or large foundations, the need for an independent organization may be more urgent than ever. One major difference between Chronic Illness Inclusion and the health organizations I have interacted with in the United States is how this new organization is devoted to including people with ELCI in all of their events including the planning phases. This type of advocacy models what is possible for other organizations while also creating a deeper understanding of how to accommodate and support the common experience of limited energy. Central to the experiences of people living with ELCI is the pattern of disbelief they encounter when communicating about their condition. In their 2020 report on chronic illness in the UK, Chronic Illness Inclusion looked at 2,300 responses to their extended qualitative forum and a follow-up survey with a focus on (1) the experiences of living with a chronic illness, (2) the barriers and ableism participants encountered, and (3) the possibilities for collective action (Hale et al., 2020). In many ways, narcolepsy has more support and treatment options than the bulk of the conditions under the umbrella of ELCI, yet in other ways, there is power in forging a shared identity and shared experiences because it has enabled significant accomplishments across the pond.

Health communication has made significant strides in the last few years in breaking patterns that may further disempower groups and individuals who may lack power in society. The growth in qualitative and rhetorical health researchers has shown traditionally quantitative health communication scholars new ways of engaging with how people communicate about health. Nevertheless, there remains a core of health communication that bases their quantitative research methods and findings on perspectives that presume that identity and culture are not at play in how individuals communicate about health and illness. Able-bodied researchers should consider supporting or collaborating with researchers who have disabilities to increase the prevalence of work that provides insight into marginalized communities.

Patient education and family education should become more of a priority for physicians and nurses who treat narcolepsy. While my research and the existence of a physician like the one the group recommended both testify to major advances in the quality of treatment and understanding of narcolepsy, these are exceptions that prove the general trend. Most of the participants in the project had physicians like the one Aurora described who knew little about the condition and, therefore, left most of the patient's education to the internet. How many families have been cast into tumult because basic information about the condition failed to reach those who need it the most? As mentioned earlier, Wolf-Meyer (2012) refers to narcoleptic patients as the model sleep patient because of their eagerness to submit to the biopolitics of surveillance and medical treatment to regain their capacity to engage with society. Medical treatment can be limited when employers, teachers, and family members can undermine treatment and behavioral adjustments because they lack the necessary education to allow them to support patients in a more productive or edifying way.

The low numbers of people who are from economically disadvantaged backgrounds in this study is not an accident, because not having access to health care or minimal access to health care might severely circumscribe their ability to get diagnosed much less participate in a project like this. Engaging people who received health insurance benefits from being on Social Security disability piques my interest in seeing more acknowledgments of health insurance status and form (public vs. private) in health communication research. The statistically significant differences in communication behaviors between uninsured people compared with insured people suggests that insurance type may similarly influence sensemaking processes (Cheong et al., 2007). As previously discussed, throughout my time in the field and while analyzing the interviews and observations, my race, socioeconomic background, sexuality, and age all influenced my experience of the research. Similarly, the intersectionality of each interviewee is a part of their story and their experience of narcolepsy. Future research on hidden disabilities may choose to focus more on the dynamics of intersectionality as it is perceived by the interviewees or the researcher. Research on neurodiversity conditions at the intersection of class and race may provide a rich account of the way ableism operates in relationship to these and other aspects of inequality. Future research on neurological conditions, autoimmune conditions, or other hidden disabilities may seek to develop an intricate way of thinking about the role of place in the experience of symptoms.

While many people with narcolepsy can, at times, be vulnerable to accusations of not being awake enough or active enough, people who are members of minority groups may lack resources and experiences that might assuage such assaults on their character. The oppression of people with disabilities and the treatment of people with chronic illnesses both unfold in a racialized and gendered world, and efforts to describe or analyze them also reflect the intersecting and interlocking structures that reify the meaning of these categories. Indictments regarding who is aware enough and who is able enough to be a citizen, a student, a parent, a worker, or even alive hinge on the way unexamined bodily norms are permitted to permeate society unabated. In the immediate future, norms about what sleep is and when it might possibly occur may continue to marginalize and discipline people who resemble my interviewees. Nevertheless, narratives of people with narcolepsy and the thankless work of other spatiotemporal rebels will continue to disseminate a vision of life that recognizes, and may even embrace, the possibility of sleeping everywhere.

NOTE

1. Berger and Luckmann (1990) claim that others' realities are characterized by modes of experience and are viewed as "an excursion" (p. 25). That is where individuals may leave their sense of reality and join someone's reality in an excursion.

Appendix

Methods for Listening to Others and Crafting Narratives

As discussed in chapter 1, one central challenge to writing about narcolepsy is the way people with narcolepsy are often partially aware of themselves while experiencing many of the symptoms that are unique to the condition. A novel methodology was needed to get around this challenge; to put interviewees' voices center stage while also allowing us to explore our shared experiences when the opportunity arose. This appendix describes many of the methodological decisions that brought the voices of others in conversation with my story about living with narcolepsy while also including demographic details about the interviewees. This research emerged as an effort to capture the relationships people with narcolepsy have with the various places where symptoms and side effects emerge. As discussed in the preface, I drew on Lindahl's (2012) peer interview model that facilitated sharing stories between the interviewer and the interviewee. The unique nature of narcolepsy and its different presentations meant developing a process of entering the field and remaining in the field that allowed ongoing flexibility on the part of the interviewees and the interviewer. Then I detail the creation of narratives from the research by drawing on autoethnography, narrative inquiry, performance studies, and sensory ethnography. Demonstrating how going into a unique terrain where there were few models of research examining race, disability, and place required making methodological innovations that inevitably influenced the way the participant narratives unfolded and how they ultimately took shape in the book.

SUPPORT GROUP PARTICIPATION

According to the group's Facebook page, Jane created the "N in Columbus" page in 2013. However, the support group existed long before Jane joined the group and eventually started running it. The original sleep disorder support group had members with narcolepsy and sleep apnea. They had the help of a psychologist, who would help organize events and meetings at a local hospital. Since sleep apnea is much more common than narcolepsy and is very different from narcolepsy, the people with narcolepsy decided to start their own group. Sable and Nancy, as discussed in chapter 5, started this other group for people with narcolepsy. They had a group of people who came and met regularly, but they had difficulty attracting new members. This was when Jane came along and started posting meetings on Facebook. In August 2013, Jane posted a potluck as the first event for the group on Facebook; twenty people were invited because only twenty people were in the Facebook group. That year the meetings were called "Monday Meetings" and they met at a coffee shop during happy hour. The Facebook presence brought people who were newly diagnosed to the meetings which is what Sable and Nancy had struggled with. The Facebook page also has moved a lot of the communication between people in the group online in the form of posts, comments, messages, and surveys—likely somewhat weakening the demand for face-to-face dialogues. As of May 2022, the group has nearly 300 members on Facebook, but during the months leading up to my interviews there were a little over 200 group members.

I initiated communication with the support group leader, Jane, and began attending meetings to get to know members and to participate. At the first meeting, I arrived a little late and met some of the members who were interviewed and others who were not interviewed. After I introduced myself and my research I participated in their conversations about medications, symptoms, and doctors. The following month, someone other than Jane posted the details for the support group meeting event on the group's Facebook page, and I indicated my intention to attend along with five others. This was my first ninety-minute trip to sit alone in the restaurant. Initially this cast doubt on the feasibility of my research goals, but I ultimately remained committed and steadfast.

The second time I drove from Athens to Columbus to find that no one showed up for the meeting I messaged Jane and told her about no one showing up. Jane apologized for that and explained how people mean well, but "we still have a big interest in the group but unfortunately are just a big group of sleepy people." Of course, my most immediate concern was whether I would be able to do interviews and participate in meetings, but I was still somewhat curious about what was happening to create this nexus. I also offered to help host meetings if she needed help. Jane added me as an administrator, meaning I could create events and add members on the Facebook page. I later learned that Jane has had transportation issues and was reticent about asking for a ride to the meetings. After getting to know the group more, and after more empty meetings, I realized what was likely going on. As discussed in chapter 1, a potential impediment for support groups for people with a debilitating sleep disorder is that members and leaders may often lack the energy or other resources needed to attend and organize the meetings. It was just as Jane said in her message to me.

Prior to the next meeting, I created a Facebook post about recruiting people with narcolepsy to interview and posted it to the group. The post linked to my personal webpage, which had a link to download the letter of invitation that included all the information necessary for informed consent. For May's meeting, I created the monthly second Saturday support group meeting event on Facebook and drove for ninety minutes, not knowing if anyone would show up or not. As detailed in chapter 3, that day I met Penny, John, Cynthia, Jane, Elaine, and Cameron. Jane did a remarkable job of making everyone feel welcome. She gave everyone multiple black elastic wrist bands that said, "make art. advocate sleep" and mini-sketch books she made herself while also sharing books and resources with the group. Later, Jane introduced me to Nancy and Sable and I met Aurora during another meeting. At the end of the summer, I had only one male participant, so I asked Nancy if she knew of other men who might be willing to meet with me. She emailed me the contact information for several men who were once more active in the group, and I interviewed Grouse and Levi. I also have collected artifacts from my time with people in the support group to help create a rich account of the place and my time there.

My involvement with the support group is one of the ways that I seek to give back to the group. But it is also a way to keep in touch with the people I interviewed to see how their lives and conditions continued to change over time. During a support group meeting I presented a general sketch of what my preliminary research looked like at that point in time. For the following year I continued to attend meetings and took a more active role in planning the meetings and although my role in the support group changed, the group's role in the project did not change. In other words, although I became central to the support group the group was not central to my research. Rather, the individuals who I met there continued to be a primary purpose of my involvement in the group. I attended a total of eleven support group meetings—for three of the meetings no others attended. After meetings, I took notes about how the meeting went, who came, and what was discussed. The meetings allowed me to make sure what I was hearing in the interviews and analysis were consistent with how others with narcolepsy were managing their daily lives.

EMBODIED AND IN SITU INTERVIEWS

I conducted a total of twenty interviews with eleven individuals with narcolepsy (see table A.1). Each participant selected the pseudonym that is used for them. The interviews ranged from thirty minutes to 131 minutes. The first interviews were conducted in a variety of locations (home of participant, at a public library, at a Starbucks, at a hotel, or at the workplace of the participant). For the second interview the range of places was slightly wider (at a church, in a car, at a library, at a workplace, at a skate park, at a dance studio, and at a restaurant). I videorecorded most of the second interviews except for Sable's interview in a car because there was no place to perch the laptop and plug it in. Four of my participants have narcolepsy with cataplexy; the remaining have narcolepsy without cataplexy. Five participants have a graduate degree and four have four-year college degrees. Eight of my interviewees are female and three are male. The average age of my participants was forty-nine years old with an average diagnosis age of thirty-three years old. The average age of onset of symptoms was twelve years old.

All the interviews began with discussing the informed consent form and letting them know that they could stop the interview or not answer questions at any time. I had them fill out a contact information form which asked them to select their pseudonym. Then, participants answered brief questions about their demographics and diagnosis story. Occasionally, I recorded this part of the interview, which allowed me to listen to how I framed the interviews and note that it usually took between ten and twenty-five minutes to get to the first interview question. Often aspects of their narcolepsy would not get recorded because they were shared before I began recording the interview and were not made explicit in the interview or paperwork. With Elaine, for example, she spoke about her current concerns at length during the pre-interview phase of our time together.

The first interviews were designed to facilitate dialogue (Lindahl, 2012), develop conversations (Brinkmann & Kavale, 2015), elicit stories (Pink, 2015), and help process my observations (Rubin & Rubin, 2012). Moreover, by seeking to coproduce utterances, I am building on one of the types of participant interviews that Brinkmann and Kavale (2015) discuss in their book on interviewing. To begin, I would discuss how there are three main questions for the interview: What is your diagnosis story? What areas of your life are most affected by narcolepsy? and What relationships help you manage narcolepsy? I also let them know that while I will take notes, I also will share

Table A.1. Participant's Demographic Information

Participant	*Number of Interviews*	*Age (Diagnosis Age)*	*Highest Education*	*Relationship Status*	*Employment Status*	*Primary Income*	*Race*
Penny*	2	29 (28)	Graduate	Married	Employed	No	White
John	2	49 (43)	College	Married	Self-employed	Yes	Black
Aurora*	2	53 (44)	Some college	Divorced	Employed	Yes	Black
Jane*	3	47 (25)	College	Single	Social Security disability	Yes	White
Sable*	2	56 (18)	Some college	Married	Disability retirement	Yes	White
Nancy*	3	77 (27)	Graduate	Married	Retired	No	White
Cynthia	2	42 (28)	College	Single	Employed	Yes	Black
Cameron	1	27 (23)	Graduate	Married	Employed	No	White
Elaine	1	35 (35)	College	Married	Employed	No	White
Grouse	1	61 (54)	Graduate	Single	Employed	Yes	White
Levi	1	66 (37)	Graduate	Married	Retired	No	White

Note: This table presents information collected from the demographic form filled out before interviews. * indicates participants with narcolepsy with cataplexy. Age refers to participants' age at time of interview, and the age they were when diagnosed is in parentheses. "Graduate" means they have a graduate degree, "College" means they finished a four-year degree, and "Some College" means they attended college but did not graduate with a four-year degree. All participant names are pseudonyms.

my experience so we can exchange stories, and at the end of the interview we will try to set up another interview. Depending on the type of conversation we were having and my attention to the interviewee, I would rephrase the questions or ask questions that were not listed on the probes to get more information or to explore a topic that was broached.

While the first interview was a semistructured interview with dozens of possible probe questions to make sure all relevant areas were covered, the second interview was an unstructured interview designed after the walking interview. The walking interview is a way of collecting stories in the contexts in which they occur (Dubé et al., 2014). They can make it easier for participants to take part in the study and can yield context-rich research interactions, while also allowing for serendipitous encounters between the interviewee and the interviewer (Dubé et al., 2014). Walking interviews allow researchers to collect information relating to participants' understanding of place (Butler & Derrett, 2014). Few researchers have examined the relationship between what is said and where it is spoken, and it is essential that researchers recognize the way place can influence what kind of stories can be told (Jones et al., 2008). Within rehabilitation and disability studies there are a number of benefits that walking interviews can provide including: (1) lending the interview a range of affordances that can alter the power dynamic between researcher and interviewee, (2) priming situational behaviors and thoughts for the interview, (3) facilitating increased performativity, and (4) engaging the interview as an embodied process (Butler & Derrett, 2014). Deciding on where the second interview would take place began by framing the second interview as an invitation to tell the story they would most like others to know about the influence of place on narcolepsy. If no suggestions were forthcoming, I would offer ideas based on the places that seemed most salient in their first interview while leaving the decision to the participant. Laura Ellingson (2012) claims that 90 percent of communication is nonverbal and urges us to remember that our self-presentation is a part of the interview experience. The video recording of the second interviews aided me in recounting the moments in the interview in a way that may capture both spoken and unspoken communication. These videos were only seen by me and will not be shared with anyone.

Identifying details (e.g., profession, background, appearance, and area of town) were judiciously changed in transcriptions and fieldnotes to protect the confidentiality of participants. The names of nonparticipants—like doctors, spouses, and pets—have also been changed to protect confidentiality. The second interviews, in general, are more relaxed because after the first one, they know a lot about me and are more open to sharing. After each interview, I filled out a participant summary form, which asked me to reflect on the interview considering the research questions that guided the initial project (Bloomberg & Volpe, 2016). I took over a hundred photographs before and after support group meetings and interviews to help recreate the sensory experiences of the interview. Moreover, I noted the weather, my transportation, sounds, smells, and tactile experiences while with the interviewee (Pink, 2009, 2015). My notes took the form of voice memos, handwritten notes, and typed notes. Lastly, I used both a primary recording device and a backup device in case something happened to the main recording.

My very first interview with support group members was an opportunity to adjust my expectations and refine the interview procedures. This interview was Cameron's and it immediately followed the support group meeting where I met the bulk of the participants. About an hour into the recorded interview, Cameron started to appear fatigued and asked to take a bathroom break. I decided to give my subsequent interviewees breaks and this improved the interviews markedly. Initially Cameron agreed to do a second interview, but she canceled and expressed reticence about inviting someone to her home because of all the undone housework evident in every room. I quickly learned that the initial plan of getting two interviews was not realistic for people like Cameron and possibly more of my participants. They simply may be too overwhelmed to carve out that much time. This also helps explain why the chapter on home is shorter than other chapters. Like Cameron, Elaine was swamped with caring for multiple young children and keeping a job while struggling with narcolepsy.

AUTOETHNOGRAPHIC VOICE

Instead of only drawing on fieldwork, or interviews exclusively, an autoethnographer can mine their own journal entries, memories, artifacts, photos, and feelings to gain insight into a subject matter that otherwise may be difficult to access through more traditional methods of research. Autoethnography is research that uses one's own life for data that can be illuminated through the application of theory. Some of the items I collected to construct the autoethnographic chapter include the Epworth sleepiness scales my doctor asked me to fill out, journal entries, audio recordings of head notes, and reflections on interviews. By focusing on specific spaces where sleepiness or other symptoms of narcolepsy arise, in my autoethnographic chapter, the vignettes provide intimate glimpses into how narcolepsy is experienced within everyday life. Writing also offers a way to map the journey I have taken with this condition alongside the voices of other passengers. Similar to Chawla's (2011) autoethnography, "Between Solids / Monologues in Brown: A Mystory Performance" which is a map of moving between geographies that mark bodies as (not) belonging or (not) desirable, my autoethnographic chapter explores identity, place, and an evolving sense of belonging that is intertwined with the experiences of narcolepsy.

There are several iterations of myself woven throughout this book and within the autoethnographic chapters. My narcolepsy changed during the years that proceeded my research, and through engaging with the support group I was introduced to a doctor who recommended doing a sleep test to better understand how my narcolepsy may have changed. Once I started taking the sleep medicine the group introduced me to, my symptoms markedly improved. I shared with those close to me that "it was like having a new brain." Similar to the way my narcolepsy transformed my emotional world I also went through many transformations in the years following my field research. My insights into how my racism, race and racial identity shaped my experiences of living with narcolepsy came after having spent time reading more about racism and after developing a relationship with a trusted psychologist.

My self-reflexive story of living with narcolepsy is integrated throughout the book in a few ways: I offer subjective descriptions that are not a part of observations or interviews; I write with an autoethnographic voice that uses narrative to support assertions and to present patterns; my accounts and feelings show up in conversation with my participants; and I have a chapter that is dedicated to my early journey with narcolepsy. As I use writing to map out the process, I am accompanied by a number of fellow voyagers who have shared their maps in the form of autoethnography. I am accompanied by Lisa Tillmann's (1996) forays into the land of bulimia. I am also joined by Rachel Alicia Griffin's (2012) "Black Feminist Autoethnography," rooted in the desire to "talk back" to systemic oppression (2012, p. 80). Nathan Hodges's (2015) "American Dental Dream," on the way bodies are marked by socioeconomic class, reminds me how to use autoethnography to present information and stories that other methods of writing and research tend to silence and undermine. Nicole Defenbaugh's (2011) book, *A Narrative Journey of the IBD Body,* maps out how to blend autoethnographic sensibilities with performance and critiques of medical practices. Together, with these maps and the guidance of others, my autoethnographic voice sought to show readers how I tended to navigate the terrain of my narcolepsy.

CRAFTING THE NARRATIVES

Performance studies is a way to bridge the space between the embodied accounts of life with narcolepsy and the goals of conducting research in a way that allows me to be a researcher who is engaged with participants in a meaningful manner during and after the interview. Performance studies offers theories, methods, objects of investigations, subjectivities, ways of writing, and ways of distributing products of research—it is a buffet. It willingly offers itself up and invites researchers to take only the parts of performance studies that will best suit their projects. As a result, for this project, performance studies inspired me to find engaging ways of writing about my experiences with narcolepsy and with my participants. It guided me to autoethnography, while also introducing me to narrative inquiry which offered a way to write about my observations and interviews. Like Christopher Poulos (2009, 2021) and other autoethnographers, I have chosen to narrate portions of interview transcriptions as conversational dialogue (Constantino, 2008; Pink, 2015). This is an effort to find a mode of narration that pulls together the sensory ethnographic notes, artifacts, recordings, observations, transcriptions, to either create a scene or support an analysis. Geertz (2001) refers to autoethnography as a blurred genre, and perhaps this book further blurs familiar modes of communicating about research. It seeks to "make a text present" by demanding the participation of the reader, and by refusing closure or categorization (Jones, 2006, p. 765). The potential overreliance on narrative hopes to further cultivate compassion and complexity in understanding both the peer research experience and narcolepsy in everyday life.

Using a case study approach of reporting research that focuses on one place and one interviewee for each chapter created an elegant overall organizing logic that facilitates both deep storytelling alongside rich descriptions of different lived experiences. Each chapter is a product of the interview logs, notes, photos, recordings, and transcriptions that were collected and analyzed. The photographs that were taken and are occasionally described attempt to enact what Pink (2009) describes as rendering complex sensory knowledge that is loyal to local participants' understanding. The interviewees' ability to select where they did their second interview allowed the ultimate themes of each chapter partly a collaboration with the participants. Pink (2009) uses the term *knowledge production* to replace what is typically labeled as analysis in qualitative research. Accordingly, the shift from background narrative to analysis narrative is subtlety noted in each chapter.

Interview transcriptions were analyzed using the interpretive phenomenological analysis (IPA), which encourages case study approaches to qualitative research. I used Jonathan Smith and Mike Osborn's (2015) chapter, "Interpretive Phenomenological Analysis" to guide my exploration of the selected interviews. According to Smith and Osborn (2015), the aim of IPA is "to explore in detail how participants are making sense of their personal and social world and the main currency for an IPA study is the meanings, particular experiences, events, states hold for participants" (p. 53). I analyzed the first interview by writing on a printed-out transcript, and for later interviews

I used Microsoft Excel and Microsoft Word. The steps of phenomenological analysis began with adding line numbers to transcriptions.

The next step was to make note of what was interesting or significant about the interview going line by line (Smith & Osborn, 2015). After going through the whole transcript, I returned to the top and began noting emerging themes with, "concise phrases which aim to capture the essential quality of what was found in the text" (Smith & Osborn, 2015, p. 68). The themes were grouped into clusters, and I created a table of themes to allow me to trace particular clusters back to parts of the transcription using the page number and line number. Finally, I organized the table to determine which themes fit with the others and which do not. Since these were fairly long interviews, the analysis focused on the categories of themes that occurred most frequently.

Each space and participant is viewed as an active participant in the scenes I crafted. In doing so, I weaved in detail from fieldnotes, observations, photographs, and other sources to create a rich and immersive story of a person with narcolepsy in a specific location. After I present each narrative, I reflected on the story of the interview by elaborating on what it reveals about narcolepsy before sharing stories from other interviewees that nuance or counter the themes in the case study. Each chapter presents an individual's relationship between place and narcolepsy while also exploring what the place means across different subjectivities.

ETHICAL CONSIDERATIONS

Credibility refers to the believability of the link between the participants and the analysis, between the interviews and the codes that emerge, and the perceived accuracy of the process and writing about it (Jensen, 2008a). The credibility of a research project rests on the project's practices to ensure a high level of consistency throughout the stages of the research project, and through the researcher's ability to communicate with readers and participants in a clear and effective manner (Jensen, 2008a). One of the ways to improve credibility is by spending time with participants (Jensen, 2008a). My ongoing relationship with the people in this project therefore strengthens the credibility of this project. I also manage credibility by including multiple angles of analysis, including member checks, and by including multiple sources of data/information and multiple techniques for data and information gathering (Ellingson, 2005; Jensen, 2008a; Lindlof & Taylor, 2011). Transferability refers to qualitative research results that can be transferred to other contexts and situations beyond the scope of this particular project (Jensen, 2008b). By striving to paint a full and rich picture of the research context, I allow readers to determine for themselves if the meanings they uncover in the thick descriptions can be transferred to another context (Jensen, 2008b, p. 886). Generally, qualitative research is conducted understanding that it lacks the epistemological requisites that allow what is uncovered in one set of circumstances to be transferable to a different set of circumstances.

This project embraces a form of pragmatic validity that evaluates studies based on the extent that they produce knowledge that leads to social change-directed actions (Lindlof & Taylor, 2011, p. 272; Miller, 2008, p. 909). Self-reflection, member checks, and continual verification of findings are a part of this project's research design that work to ensure a high level of validity. As an insider, I may never leave "the field" and will likely not be taxed by the burden of negotiating a complete exit. I engaged participants as both a peer and a researcher, and that relationship will be sustained far beyond the duration of this project and its discursive iterations.

References

Adams, T. E. (2006). Seeking father: Relationally reframing a troubled love story. *Qualitative Inquiry*, *12*(4), 704–723. https://doi.org/10.1177/1077800406288607

American Academy of Sleep Medicine. (2014). *International classification of sleep disorders*. American Academy of Sleep Medicine.

Andrews, M. (2014). *Narrative imagination and everyday life*. Oxford University Press.

Antonoff, J. (2013). *Brave* [Recorded by S. Bareilles]. Sony/ATV Music Publishing LLC.

Armstrong, T. (2010). *Neurodiversity: Discovering the extraordinary gifts of autism, ADHD, dyslexia, and other brain differences*. Da Capo.

Associated Press. (2014, June 20). *Court overturns law that bans people from sleeping in cars*. *NY Daily News*. http://www.nydailynews.com/news/national/court-overturns-law-bans-people-sleeping-cars-article-1.1837189

Baglieri, S., Valle, J. W., Connor, D. J., & Gallagher, D. J. (2011). Disability studies in education: The need for a plurality of perspectives on disability. *Remedial and Special Education*, *32*(4), 267–278. https://doi.org/10.1177/0741932510362200

Bailey, M. (2017, November 9). Race and Disability in the Academy. *The Sociological Review Blog*. https://www.thesociologicalreview.com/blog/race-and-disability-in-the-academy.html?utm_content=buffer3cd7c&utm_medium=social&utm_source=twitter.com&utm_campaign=buffer

Baiocchi-Wagner, E. (2011). When obesity is a crime: Family communication and individual member health. In M. Brann (Ed.), *Contemporary case studies in health communication: Theoretical & applied approaches*. Kendall Hunt.

Baker, D. L. (2011). *The politics of neurodiversity: Why public policy matters*. Lynne Rienner.

Bakhtin, M. (1987). *The dialogic imagination: Four essays* (V. N. Volochinov, Trans.). University of Texas Press.

Barbero, L., Govi, A., Pizza, F., Plazzi, G., & Ingravallo, F. (2017). Parental fitness questioned on the grounds of narcolepsy: Presentation of two cases. *Journal of Clinical Sleep Medicine*, *13*(08), 1017–1018. https://doi.org/10.5664/jcsm.6708

Barker, C. I. S., & Snape, M. D. (2014). Pandemic influenza A H1N1 vaccines and narcolepsy: Vaccine safety surveillance in action. *Lancet Infectious Diseases, 14*(3), 227–238. https://doi.org/10.1016/S1473-3099(13)70238-X

Barrett, D. (2001). *The committee of sleep: How artists, scientists, and athletes use dreams for creative problem-solving—and how you can too*. Crown Publishers.

Baum, L. F. (1900). *The wonderful wizard of Oz*. Geo M Hill Co. http://etext.lib.virginia.edu/modeng/modengB.browse.html

Bayon, V., Léger, D., & Philip, P. (2009). Socio-professional handicap and accidental risk in patients with hypersomnias of central origin. *Sleep Medicine Reviews*, *13*(6), 421–426. https://doi.org/10.1016/j.smrv.2009.02.001

Bell, C. M. (Ed.). (2011). Introduction: Doing repersentational detective work. In *Blackness and disability: Critical examinations and cultural interventions* (pp. 1–8). Michigan State University Press.

Berger, P. L., & Luckmann, T. (1990). *The social construction of reality: A treatise in the sociology of knowledge*. Anchor Books.

Bijsterveld, K., Cleophas, E., Krebs, S., & Mom, G. (2013). *Sound and safe: A history of listening behind the wheel*. Oxford University Press.

Black, J., Reaven, N. L., Funk, S. E., McGaughey, K., Ohayon, M., Guilleminault, C., Ruoff, C., & Mignot, E. (2014). The burden of narcolepsy disease (BOND) study: Health-care utilization and cost findings. *Sleep Medicine*, *15*(5), 522–529. https://doi.org/10.1016/j.sleep.2014.02.001

Bloomberg, L. D., & Volpe, M. (2016). *Completing your qualitative dissertation: A road map from beginning to end* (3rd ed.). Sage.

Boylorn, R. M. (2017). *Sweetwater: Black women and narratives of resilience* (Revised edition). Peter Lang.

Brinkmann, S., & Kavale, S. (2015). *InterViews: Learning the craft of qualitative research interviewing* (3rd ed.). Sage.

Broderick, M. L. (2016). Home birth: The wholeness of absence. *Health Communication, 31*(3), 379–381. https://doi.org/10.1080/10410236.2014.950928

Brody, J. E. (1994, April 24). America's Falling Asleep. *The New York Times*. http://www.nytimes.com/1994/04/24/magazine/good-health-america-s-falling-asleep.html

Broekhuis, M., van Velsen, L., De Franco, D., Pease, A., & Hermens, H. (2022). Contextual health information behavior in the daily lives of people with type 2 diabetes: A diary study in Scotland. *Health Communication*, *37*(3), 272–284. https://doi.org/10.1080/10410236.2020.1837426

Brooks, D. (2013). *Succeeding with Narcolepsy*. Succeeding with Narcolepsy. https://www.succeedingwithnarcolepsy.com

Brown, K. (2019). *The pretty one: On life, pop culture, disability, and other reasons to fall in love with me*. Atria.

Bruder, J. (2017). *Nomadland: Surviving America in the twenty-first century* (1st ed.). W. W. Norton & Company.

Burger, A. (2012). *The Wizard of Oz as American myth: A critical study of six versions of the story, 1900–2007*. McFarland & Co.

Butler, M., & Derrett, S. (2014). The walking interview: An ethnographic approach to understanding disability. *Internet Journal of Allied Health Sciences & Practice*, *12*(3), 1–8.

Carey, J. A. (2013). Sociopolitical contexts of passing and intellectual disability. In J. A. Brune & D. J. Wilson (Eds.), *Disability and passing: Blurring the lines of identity* (pp. 142–166). Temple University Press.

Chaudhry, B. (2017). World Day of Remembrance (November 19). *World Day of Rememberance*. http://worlddayofremembrance.org/

Chawla, D. (2011). Between solids/monologues in Brown: A Mystory performance. *Cultural Studies <=> Critical Methodologies*, *11*(1), 47–58. https://doi.org/10.1177/1532708610386921

Charon, R. (2006). *Narrative medicine: Honoring the stories of illness*. New York and Oxford: Oxford University Press.

Chawla, D. (2014). Performing home/storying selves: Home and/as identity in oral histories or refugees in India's partition. In N. Bardhan, M. P. Orbe, & B. J. Allen (Eds.), *Identity research and communication: Intercultural reflections and future directions*. Lexington Books.

Cheong, P. H., Feeley, T. H., & Servoss, T. (2007). Understanding health inequalities for uninsured Americans: A population-wide survey. *Journal of Health Communication*, *12*(3), 285–300. https://doi.org/10.1080/10810730701266430

Chesler, P. (2005). *Women and madness* (revised and updated). Palgrave Macmillan.

Cockayne, D. (2021). The feminist economic geographies of working from home and "digital by default" in Canada before, during, and after COVID-19. *Canadian Geographer, 65*(4), 499–511.

Cohen, A. (2014, July 24). *The Trendiest Law in America May Be a Ban on Sleeping in Cars*. Next City. https://nextcity.org/daily/entry/10-facts-homelessness-2014

Cohen, C. (2015). *Head case: My brain and other wonders* (First edition). Henry Holt and Company.

Cohen, F. L., & Mudro, R. W. (1992). Social distance from persons with narcolepsy and other conditions. *Loss, Grief & Care*, *5*(3–4), 61–69.

Collins, P. H. (1986). Learning from the outsider within: The sociological significance of black feminist thought. *Social Problems*, *6*, S14.

Conquergood, D. (2002). Performance studies: Interventions and radical research. *The Drama Review*, *42*(2), 145–156.

Constantino, T. (2008). Dialogue. In L. M. Given (Ed.), *The Sage encyclopedia of qualitative research methods* (pp. 212–213). Sage.

Coren, S. (2014). *Sleep thieves: An eye-opening exploration into the science and myteries of sleep*. Free Press.

Cox, P. (2013). Passing as sane, or how to get people to sit next to you on the bus. In J. A. Brune & D. J. Wilson (Eds.), *Disability and passing: Blurring the lines of identity* (pp. 99–110). Temple University Press.

Crary, J. (2013). *24/7: Late capitalism and the ends of sleep*. Verso.

Crewe, S. E. (2007). Harriet Tubman's last work: The Harriet Tubman Home for Aged and Indigent Negroes. *Journal of Gerontological Social Work*, *49*(3), 229–244. https://doi.org/10.1300/J083v49n03_13

Dauvilliers, Y. (2007). Narcolepsy with cataplexy: Hypocretin and immunological aspects. In *Neuroimmunology of Sleep* (pp. 337–352). Springer. http://link.springer.com/chapter/10.1007/978-0-387-69146-6_20

Dauvilliers, Y., Arnulf, I., & Mignot, E. (n.d.). Narcolepsy with cataplexy. *The Lancet, 369*(9560), 499–511. https://doi.org/10.1016/S0140-6736(07)60237-2

Davis, L. J. (2006). The end of identity politics and the beginning of dismodernism. In *The disability studies reader* (2nd ed., pp. 161–172). Routledge.

Defenbaugh, N. L. (2011). *Dirty tale: A narrative journey of the IBD body*. Hampton Press.

Dehaene, S. (2014). *Consciousness and the brain: Deciphering how the brain codes our thoughts*. Viking.

Dement, W. C. (1999). *The promise of sleep: A pioneer in Sleep Medicine explores the vital connection between health, happiness, and a good night's sleep*. Delacorte.

Denzin, N. K. (2003). *Performance ethnography*. Sage. http://srmo.sagepub.com/view/performance-ethnography/SAGE.xml

Diaz, J. (2001). A dream and a nightmare. *Golf Digest*, *52*(11), 90.

Dobosz, D., Gierczyk, M., & Hornby, G. (2023). Parental perspectives of home-schooling of children with special educational needs and disabilities during the COVID-19 pandemic: A review. *Journal of Research in Special Educational Needs*, *23*(1), 3–11.

Dokumaci, A. (2014). Performance as evidence in chronic disease: Measuring health status and treatment outcomes through the quantification of performance. Performance Research, 19(4), 14–23. https://doi.org/10.1080/13528165.2014.947122

Donjacour, C. E., Mets, M. A., & Verster, J. C. (2010). Narcolepsy, driving and traffic safety. In M. Goswami, S. R. Pandi-Perumal, & M. J. Thorpy (Eds.), *Narcolepsy* (pp. 217–221). Springer. https://doi.org/10.1007/978-1-4419-0854-4_19

Doshi, M. J. (2014). Help(less): An autoethnography about caring for my mother with terminal cancer. *Health Communication*, *29*(8), 840–842. https://doi.org/10.1080/10410236.2013.809502

Du Bois, W. E. B. (1903). The talented tenth. In B. T. Washington (Ed.), *The Negro problem: A series of articles by representative American Negroes of today* (pp. 31–76). J. Pott.

Dubé, T. V., Schinke, R. J., Strasser, R., & Lightfoot, N. (2014). Interviewing in situ: Employing the guided walk as a dynamic form of qualitative inquiry. *Medical Education*, *48*(11), 1092–1100. https://doi.org/10.1111/medu.12532

Ekirch, A. R. (2006). *At day's close: Night in times past*. Norton.

Ellingson, L. L. (2005). *Communicating in the clinic: Negotiating frontstage and backstage teamwork*. Hampton.

Ellingson, L. L. (2012). Interview as embodied communication. In J. F. Gubrium (Ed.), *The Sage handbook of interview research: The complexity of the craft* (2nd ed., pp. 525–540). Sage.

Epilepsy Foundation. (n.d.). *Driving and epilepsy—A study regarding car accidents and seizure as cause*. Epilepsy Foundation. Retrieved May 23, 2017, from http:

//www.epilepsy.com/connect/forums/living-epilepsy-adults/driving-and-epilepsy-study-regarding-car-accidents-and-seizure

Eugene, N. (2006). Bridges of Katrina: Three survivors, one interview. *Callaloo*, *29*(4), 1507–1512.

Eugene, N. (2013). Working while narcoleptic. *Anthropology of Consciousness*, *24*(2), 158–171.

Eugene, N. (2017). (Un)becoming mistakes [poem]. In D. A. Ryskamp & S. Harvey (Eds.), *The spoon knife anthology (book 2)* (p. 78). NeuroQueer Books.

Eyler, J. R. (2013). Disability and prosthesis in L. Frank Baum's *The Wonderful Wizard of Oz*. *Children's Literature Association Quarterly*, *38*(3), 319–334. https://doi.org/10.1353/chq.2013.0042

Falvo, D. (2009). *Medical and psychosocial aspects of chronic illness and disability*. Omnigraphics.

Fitzsimmons, E. G. (2016, November 16). Engineer in Hoboken Train Crash Had Undiagnosed Sleep Disorder, Lawyer Says. *The New York Times*. https://www.nytimes.com/2016/11/17/nyregion/engineer-in-hoboken-train-crash-had-undiagnosed-sleep-disorder-lawyer-says.html

Fleetwood, J. (2017). Public health, ethics, and autonomous vehicles. *American Journal of Public Health*, *107*(4), 632–537.

Flores, N. M., Villa, K. F., Black, J., Chervin, R. D., & Witt, E. A. (2016). The humanistic and economic burden of narcolepsy. *Journal Of Clinical Sleep Medicine*, *12*(3), 401–407. https://doi.org/10.5664/jcsm.5594

Flygare, J. (2013). *Wide awake and dreaming: A memoir of narcolepsy*. Mill Pond Swan.

Flygare, J. (2014, November 9). *Watch Now: How a Patient Helped Define A New Clinical Endpoint with FDA* [Blog]. JulieFlygare.Com. http://julieflygare.com/watch-now-how-a-patient-helped-define-a-new-clinical-endpoint-with-fda/

Frank, A. W. (1995). *The wounded storyteller: Body, illness, and ethics / Arthur W Frank*. University of Chicago Press.

Garland-Thomson, R. (2011). Misfits: A feminist materialist disability conc *Hypatia*, *26*(3), 591–609.

Garland-Thomson, R. (2014). The story of my work: How I became disa *Disability Studies Quarterly*, *34*(2), 8–8. https://doi.org/10.18061/dsq.v34i2.4

Geertz, C. (2001). *Local knowledge: Further essays in interpretive anthropolog* ed.). Basic Books.

Glennon, A. M. (2017, March). *Medusa in Ancient Greek Art | Essay Metropolitan Museum of Art | Heilbrunn Timeline of Art History*. Th Heilbrunn Timeline of Art History. https://www.metmuseum.org/toah/ hd_medu.htm

Goffman, E. (2006). Selections from Stigma. In L. J. Davis (Ed.), *The disa ies reader* (2nd ed, pp. 131–140). Routledge.

Grandner, M. A., Williams, N. J., Knutson, K. L., Roberts, D., & G. (2016). Sleep disparity, race/ethnicity, and socioeconomic po *Medicine*, *18*, 7–18. https://doi.org/10.1016/j.sleep.2015.01.020

Grealy, L. (2016). *Autobiography of a face*. Harper Collins.

Griffin, R. A. (2012). I AM an angry Black woman: Black feminist autoethnography, voice, and resistance. *Women's Studies in Communication*, *35*(2), 138–157. https://doi.org/10.1080/07491409.2012.724524

Gross, T., & Kimmel, J. (Directors). (2013). Jimmy Kimmel on dealing with Narcolepsy. In *Fresh Air*. https://soundcloud.com/freshair/jimmy-kimmel-on-dealing-with

Guturu, H., Chinchali, S., Clarke, S. L., & Bejerano, G. (2016). Erosion of conserved binding sites in personal genomes points to medical histories. *PLOS Computational Biology*, *12*(2), e1004711. https://doi.org/10.1371/journal.pcbi.1004711

Hale, C., Benstead, S., Lyus, J., Odell, E., & Ruddock, A. (2020). *Energy Impairment and Disability Inclusion*. Center for Welfare Reform. https://chronicillnessinclusion.org.uk/wp-content/uploads/2021/04/energy-impairment-and-disability-inclusion.pdf

Haller, B. (2004). Wicked. *Disability Studies Quarterly*, *24*(2). http://dsq-sds.org/article/view/495

Haltom, B. (2015). A supreme nap. *Tennessee Bar Journal*, *51*(4), 40–41.

Haraway, D. (1999). A cyborg manifesto. In S. During (Ed.), *The cultural studies reader* (2nd ed., pp. 271–291). Routledge.

…ht, M. L., Jackson, R. L., & Ribeau, S. A. (2003). *African American communica-…n: Exploring identity and culture* (2nd ed.). L. Erlbaum Associates.

… M. (2009, April 9). Going to church. *Forbes*, *183*(8), 20–22.

…an, J. M. (2012). *Black and blue: The origins and consequences of medical …* University of California Press.

… (2015). The American dental dream. *Health Communication*, *30*(9), …ttps://doi.org/10.1080/10410236.2014.914621

…997). Talking back. In J. O'Brien & P. Kollock (Eds.), *The production …* 546–549). Sage.

… (2016). *The sleep revolution: Transforming your life, one night at …* Books.

…i, V., Pizza, F., Vignatelli, L., Govi, A., Dormi, A., Pelotti, S., …illiers, Y., & Plazzi, G. (2012). The burden of narcolepsy with …se history and clinical features influence socio-economic out-…*e*, *13*(10), 1293–1300. https://doi.org/10.1016/j.sleep.2012…

…way Safety. (2017, April). *Safety belts*. IIHS. http://www…afetybeltuse?topicName=Safety%20belts#tableData

…erglund, B. (2015). Participation in society for people …*bility and Health Journal*, *8*(1), 44–50. https://doi.org…

…yism and the health of African-Americans. *Culture,* …), 163–182. https://doi.org/10.1007/BF01379448

…). Desperately seeking legitimacy: Narratives of a …In L. M. Harter, P. M. Japp, & C. S. Beck (Eds.), …*Communication theory, research and practice* (pp. …ciates.

Jensen, D. (2008a). Credibility. In L. M. Given (Ed.), *The Sage encyclopedia of qualitative research methods* (Vols. 1 & 2, pp. 138–139). Sage.

Jensen, D. (2008b). Transferability. In L. M. Given (Ed.), *The Sage encyclopedia of qualitative research methods* (Vols. 1 & 2, p. 886). Sage.

Johnson, B. D. (2017). Brave new road. *Mechanical Engineering-CIME, 3*, 30–36. edsgao.

Jones, J. L. (2006). Performance and ethnography, performing ethnography, performance ethnography. In D. S. Madison & J. Hamera (Eds.), *The Sage handbook of performance studies* (pp. 339–364). Sage.

Jones, P., Bunce, G., Evans, J., Gibbs, H., & Hein, J. R. (2008). Exploring space and place with walking interviews. *Journal of Research Practice*, *4*(2), 1–9.

Julian, R. (1998). "I love driving": Alternative constructions of Hmong femininity in the West. *Race, Gender & Class*, *5*(2), 30–53.

Kafer, A. (2013). *Feminist, queer, crip*. Indiana University Press.

Kapella, M. C., Berger, B. E., Vern, B. A., Vispute, S., Prasad, B., & Carley, D. W. (2015). Health-related stigma as a determinant of functioning in young adults with narcolepsy. *PLoS ONE*, *10*(4), e0122478. PMC. https://doi.org/10.1371/journal.pone.0122478

Kendi, I. X. (2016). *Stamped from the beginning: The definitive history of racist ideas in America*. Nation Books.

Kendi, I. X. (2019). *How to be an antiracist*. One World.

Kleinman, A. (1989). *The illness narratives: Suffering, healing, and the human condition*. Basic Books.

Krahn, L. E., Lymp, J. F., Moore, W. R., Slocumb, N., & Silber, M. H. (2005). Characterizing the emotions that trigger cataplexy. *The Journal of Neuropsychiatry and Clinical Neurosciences*, *17*(1), 45–50.

Kramer, K. (2009). Shifting and seizing: A call to reform Ohio's outdated restrictions on drivers with epilepsy. *Journal of Law and Health*, *22*(2), 343–374.

Kreps, G. L. (2006). Communication and racial inequities in health care. *American Behavioral Scientist*, *49*(6), 760–774. https://doi.org/10.1177/0002764205283800

Kroker, K. (2007). *The sleep of others and the transformations of sleep research*. University of Toronto Press.

Kryger, M. H., Walld, R., & Manfreda, J. (2002). Diagnoses received by narcolepsy patients in the year prior to diagnosis by a sleep specialist. *Sleep*, *25*(1), 36–41. https://doi.org/10.1093/sleep/25.1.36

Laderman, D. (2002). *Driving visions: Exploring the road movie* (1st ed.). University of Texas Press.

Lambert, G. (2021, July 17). *The woman who "lies on the floor" to highlight her disability*. BristolLive. https://www.bristolpost.co.uk/news/bristol-news/woman-chronic-pain-who-lies-5605836

Langellier, K. M. (1999). Personal narrative, performance, performativity: Two or three things I know for sure. *Text and Performance Quarterly*, *19*(2), 125–144. https://doi.org/10.1080/10462939909366255

Laymon, K. (2018). *Heavy: An American memoir* (1st ed.). Scribner.

Lee, L., & Molnar, F. (2017). Driving and dementia. [Abstract]. *Canadian Family Physician*, *63*(1), 27–31.

Lewis, M. (1997, September 21). Bill Clinton's Garbage Man. *The New York Times*, 58.

Lezotte, C. (2015). Women Auto Know: Automotive knowledge, auto activism, and women's online car advice. *Feminist Media Studies*, *15*(4), 691–706. https://doi.org/10.1080/14680777.2014.987151

Liguori, C., Izzi, F., Mercuri, N. B., Tarantino, U., & Placidi, F. (2017). Physical activity contradictorily affects bone mineral density in obstructive sleep apnea patients at different ages. [Letter to the Editor]. *Sleep Medicine*, *32*, 273. https://doi.org/10.1016/j.sleep.2016.09.024

Lindahl, C. (2006). Survivor to survivor: Katrina stories from Houston: Recording Katrina: The survivor duet. *Callaloo*, *29*(4), 1506–1507.

Lindahl, C. (2012). Legends of hurricane Katrina: The right to be wrong, survivor-to-survivor storytelling, and healing. *Journal of American Folklore*, *125*(496), 139–178. Literature Resource Center.

Lindahl, C., Baddeley, J., Nash, S., Smothers, S., Eugene, N., & Mcfadden, V. (2009). Archiving the voices and needs of Katrina's children: The uses and importance of stories narrated survivor-to-survivor. *Children, Law, and Disasters: What We Have Learned from the Hurricanes oOf 2005*, 61–112.

Lindlof, T. R., & Taylor, B. C. (2011). *Qualitative communication research methods* (3rd ed.). Sage.

Loewit-Phillips, P. M., & Goldbas, A. (2013). Mothers Against Drunk Driving (MADD): History and impact. *International Journal of Childbirth Education*, *28*(4), 62–67.

Lundgren, B. (2015). Narrating narcolepsy—Centering a side effect. *Medical Anthropology*, *34*(2), 150–165. https://doi.org/10.1080/01459740.2014.962694

Macy, B. (2018). *Dopesick: Dealers, doctors, and the drug company that addicted America* (1st ed.). Little, Brown and Company.

Marín Agudelo, H. A., Jiménez Correa, U., Carlos Sierra, J., Pandi-Perumal, S. R., & Schenck, C. H. (2014). Cognitive behavioral treatment for narcolepsy: Can it complement pharmacotherapy? *Sleep Science*, *7*(1), 30–42. https://doi.org/10.1016/j.slsci.2014.07.023

Mayer, G., Bassetti, C. L., & Dauvilliers, Y. (2013). Treatment options in narcolepsy. *Expert Opinion on Orphan Drugs*, *1*(12), 987–999. https://doi.org/10.1517/21678707.2013.854701

Mazzetti, M., Bellucci, C., Mattarozzi, K., Plazzi, G., Tuozzi, G., & Cipolli, C. (2010). REM-dreams recall in patients with narcolepsy-cataplexy. [Abstract]. *Brain Research Bulletin*, *81*(1), 133–140. https://doi.org/doi:10.1016/j.brainresbull.2009.10.021

McCall, C. A., & Watson, N. F. (2020). Therapeutic strategies for mitigating driving risk in patients with narcolepsy. *Therapeutics and Clinical Risk Management*, *Volume 16*, 1099–1108. https://doi.org/10.2147/TCRM.S244714

McGhee, H. C. (2021). *The sum of us: What racism costs everyone and how we can prosper together* (1st ed.). One World.

Mehan, H. (2010). Five features of reality. In J. O'Brien (Ed.), *The production of reality: Essays and readings on social interaction* (5th ed., pp. 363–379). Pine Forge.

Merritt, S. L. (2004). *Mood, perceived stigma and health status self-disclosures of young adults with narcolepsy. 27.* http://www.journalsleep.org/PDF/AbstractBook2004.pdf

Merritt, S. L., Cohen, F. L., & Smith, K. M. (1992). Learning style preferences of persons with narcolepsy. In M. Goswami (Ed.), *Psychosocial aspects of narcolepsy* (pp. 115–127). Haworth.

Meskill, G. J., Kallweit, U., Zarycranski, D., Caussé, C., Finance, O., Ligneau, X., & Davis, C. W. (2021). Pitolisant for the treatment of cataplexy in adults with narcolepsy. *Expert Opinion on Orphan Drugs*, *9*(11–12), 237–246. https://doi.org/10.1080/21678707.2021.2022472

Mets, M. A. J., Alford, C., & Verster, J. C. (2012). Sleep specialists' opinion on sleep disorders and fitness to drive a car: The necessity of continued education. *Industrial Health*, *50*(6), 499–508.

Miller, P. (2008). Validity. In L. M. Given (Ed.), *The Sage encyclopedia of qualitative research methods* (Vols. 1 & 2, pp. 909–910). Sage.

Moore, L. (2020, June 22). *When Can We Come Home? Healing Open Wounds of Black Ableism By Speaking Black Disabled Ancestors Through Poetry & Introducing Krip-Hop Politics*. Academics for Black Survival and Wellness, Online.

Morandin, M., & Bruck, D. (2013). Understanding automatic behavior in narcolepsy: New insights using a phenomenological approach. [Abstract]. *The Open Sleep Journal*, *6*(1), 1–7.

National Sleep Foundation. (2012). *2012 Sleep in America Poll: Planes, Trains and Automobiles* (p. 83) [Summary of Findings]. The National Sleep Foundation. http: www.sleepfoundation.org/2012pol

National Sleep Foundation. (2017). *Facts and Stats: Drowsy Driving—Stay Alert, Arrive Alive*. DrowsyDriving.Org. http://drowsydriving.org/about/facts-and-stats/

Naumann, A., Bellebaum, C., & Daum, I. (2006). Cognitive deficits in narcolepsy. *Journal of Sleep Research*, *15*(3), 329–338. https://doi.org/10.1111/j.1365–2869.2006.00533.x

Nero, C. I. (2016). Black queer identity, imaginative rationality, and the language of home. In A. González & Y.-W. Chen (Eds.), *Our voices: Essays in culture, ethnicity, and communication* (6th ed.). Oxford University Press.

Nicholls, H. (2018). *Sleepy head: Narcolepsy, neuroscience and the search for a good night*. Basic Books.

Obasogie, O. K., & Newman, Z. (2016). Black Lives Matter and respectability politics in local news accounts of officer-involved civilian deaths: An early empirical assessment. *Wisconsin Law Review*, *2016*(3), 541–574.

Ohayon, M. M. (2013). Narcolepsy is complicated by high medical and psychiatric comorbidities: A comparison with the general population. *Sleep Medicine*, *14*(6), 488–492. https://doi.org/10.1016/j.sleep.2013.03.002

Okello, W. K. (2021). Organized anxiety: Respectability politics, John Henryism, and the paradox of Black achievement. *Race, Ethnicity & Education*, *24*(4), 523–541.

Onion, R. (2015). Driving off into the sunset: The California street-racing and the mobile-DJ scenes. *The Virginia Quarterly Review*, *3*, 275–278.

Opie, J. (2009). Naps for invention. *Wilson Quarterly*, *33*(1), 81–81.

O'Rourke, M. (2022). *The invisible kingdom: Reimagining chronic illness*. Riverhead Books.

Our history. (2018). Chronic Illness Inclusion. https://chronicillnessinclusion.org.uk/our-history/

Pachana, N. A., Jetten, J., Gustafsson, L., & Liddle, J. (2016). To be or not to be (an older driver): Social identity theory and driving cessation in later life. [Abstract]. *Ageing and Society*, 1–12. https://doi.org/10.1017/S0144686X16000507

Pelias, R. J. (2019). *The creative qualitative researcher: Writing that makes readers want to read*. Routledge.

Pfuetze, P. (1961). *Self, society, existence: Human nature and dialogue in the thought of George Herbert Mead and Martin Buber* (2nd ed.). Torchbooks.

Philip, P., Chaufton, C., Taillard, J., Sagaspe, P., Léger, D., Raimondi, M., Vakulin, A., & Capelli, A. (2013). Maintenance of Wakefulness Test scores and driving performance in sleep disorder patients and controls. *International Journal of Psychophysiology*, *89*(2), 195–202. https://doi.org/10.1016/j.ijpsycho.2013.05.013

Philip, P., Sagaspe, P., Lagarde, E., Leger, D., Ohayon, M. M., Bioulac, B., Boussuge, J., & Taillard, J. (2010). Sleep disorders and accidental risk in a large group of regular registered highway drivers. [Abstract]. *Sleep Medicine*, *11*(10), 973–979. https://doi.org/10.1016/j.sleep.2010.07.010

Phillips, R. O., & Sagberg, F. (2013). Road accidents caused by sleepy drivers: Update of a Norwegian survey. [Abstract]. *Accident Analysis & Prevention*, *50*, 138–146. https://doi.org/10.1016/j.aap.2012.04.003

Pink, S. (2009). *Doing sensory ethnography* (1st ed.). Sage.

Pink, S. (2015). *Doing sensory ethnography* (2nd ed.). Sage.

Plazzi, G. (2013). Dante's description of narcolepsy. *Sleep Medicine*, *14*(11), 1221–1223. https://doi.org/10.1016/j.sleep.2013.07.005

Potenza, A. (2013). The end of America's car culture? Once a symbol of the American dream and young adulthood, cars seem to be losing some of their appeal. *New York Times Upfront*, *3*, 10.

Poulos, C. N. (2009). *Accidental ethnography: An inquiry into family secrecy*. Left Coast.

Poulos, C. N. (2021). *Essentials of autoethnography*. American Psychological Association.

Presswood, A. L. (2020). *Food blogs, postfeminism, and the communication of expertise: Digital domestics*. Lexington Books.

Price, D. (2021). *Laziness does not exist: A defense of the exhausted, exploited, and overworked*. Atria Books.

Project Sleep. (n.d.). *Narcolepsy: Not alone*. NARCOLEPSY: NOT ALONE (TM). http://narcolepsynotalone.com/

Richardson, L. (1997). *Fields of play: Constructing an academic life*. Rutgers University Press.

//www.epilepsy.com/connect/forums/living-epilepsy-adults/driving-and-epilepsy-study-regarding-car-accidents-and-seizure

Eugene, N. (2006). Bridges of Katrina: Three survivors, one interview. *Callaloo, 29*(4), 1507–1512.

Eugene, N. (2013). Working while narcoleptic. *Anthropology of Consciousness, 24*(2), 158–171.

Eugene, N. (2017). (Un)becoming mistakes [poem]. In D. A. Ryskamp & S. Harvey (Eds.), *The spoon knife anthology (book 2)* (p. 78). NeuroQueer Books.

Eyler, J. R. (2013). Disability and prosthesis in L. Frank Baum's *The Wonderful Wizard of Oz. Children's Literature Association Quarterly, 38*(3), 319–334. https://doi.org/10.1353/chq.2013.0042

Falvo, D. (2009). *Medical and psychosocial aspects of chronic illness and disability*. Omnigraphics.

Fitzsimmons, E. G. (2016, November 16). Engineer in Hoboken Train Crash Had Undiagnosed Sleep Disorder, Lawyer Says. *The New York Times*. https://www.nytimes.com/2016/11/17/nyregion/engineer-in-hoboken-train-crash-had-undiagnosed-sleep-disorder-lawyer-says.html

Fleetwood, J. (2017). Public health, ethics, and autonomous vehicles. *American Journal of Public Health, 107*(4), 632–537.

Flores, N. M., Villa, K. F., Black, J., Chervin, R. D., & Witt, E. A. (2016). The humanistic and economic burden of narcolepsy. *Journal Of Clinical Sleep Medicine, 12*(3), 401–407. https://doi.org/10.5664/jcsm.5594

Flygare, J. (2013). *Wide awake and dreaming: A memoir of narcolepsy*. Mill Pond Swan.

Flygare, J. (2014, November 9). *Watch Now: How a Patient Helped Define A New Clinical Endpoint with FDA* [Blog]. JulieFlygare.Com. http://julieflygare.com/watch-now-how-a-patient-helped-define-a-new-clinical-endpoint-with-fda/

Frank, A. W. (1995). *The wounded storyteller: Body, illness, and ethics / Arthur W. Frank.* University of Chicago Press.

Garland-Thomson, R. (2011). Misfits: A feminist materialist disability concept. *Hypatia, 26*(3), 591–609.

Garland-Thomson, R. (2014). The story of my work: How I became disabled. *Disability Studies Quarterly, 34*(2), 8–8. https://doi.org/10.18061/dsq.v34i2.4254

Geertz, C. (2001). *Local knowledge: Further essays in interpretive anthropology* (3rd ed.). Basic Books.

Glennon, A. M. (2017, March). *Medusa in Ancient Greek Art | Essay | The Metropolitan Museum of Art | Heilbrunn Timeline of Art History*. The Met's Heilbrunn Timeline of Art History. https://www.metmuseum.org/toah/hd/medu/hd_medu.htm

Goffman, E. (2006). Selections from Stigma. In L. J. Davis (Ed.), *The disability studies reader* (2nd ed, pp. 131–140). Routledge.

Grandner, M. A., Williams, N. J., Knutson, K. L., Roberts, D., & Jean-Louis, G. (2016). Sleep disparity, race/ethnicity, and socioeconomic position. *Sleep Medicine, 18*, 7–18. https://doi.org/10.1016/j.sleep.2015.01.020

Grealy, L. (2016). *Autobiography of a face*. Harper Collins.

Griffin, R. A. (2012). I AM an angry Black woman: Black feminist autoethnography, voice, and resistance. *Women's Studies in Communication*, *35*(2), 138–157. https://doi.org/10.1080/07491409.2012.724524

Gross, T., & Kimmel, J. (Directors). (2013). Jimmy Kimmel on dealing with Narcolepsy. In *Fresh Air*. https://soundcloud.com/freshair/jimmy-kimmel-on-dealing-with

Guturu, H., Chinchali, S., Clarke, S. L., & Bejerano, G. (2016). Erosion of conserved binding sites in personal genomes points to medical histories. *PLOS Computational Biology*, *12*(2), e1004711. https://doi.org/10.1371/journal.pcbi.1004711

Hale, C., Benstead, S., Lyus, J., Odell, E., & Ruddock, A. (2020). *Energy Impairment and Disability Inclusion*. Center for Welfare Reform. https://chronicillnessinclusion.org.uk/wp-content/uploads/2021/04/energy-impairment-and-disability-inclusion.pdf

Haller, B. (2004). Wicked. *Disability Studies Quarterly*, *24*(2). http://dsq-sds.org/article/view/495

Haltom, B. (2015). A supreme nap. *Tennessee Bar Journal*, *51*(4), 40–41.

Haraway, D. (1999). A cyborg manifesto. In S. During (Ed.), *The cultural studies reader* (2nd ed., pp. 271–291). Routledge.

Hecht, M. L., Jackson, R. L., & Ribeau, S. A. (2003). *African American communication: Exploring identity and culture* (2nd ed.). L. Erlbaum Associates.

Herper, M. (2009, April 9). Going to church. *Forbes*, *183*(8), 20–22.

Hoberman, J. M. (2012). *Black and blue: The origins and consequences of medical racism*. University of California Press.

Hodges, N. (2015). The American dental dream. *Health Communication*, *30*(9), 943–950. https://doi.org/10.1080/10410236.2014.914621

hooks, bell. (1997). Talking back. In J. O'Brien & P. Kollock (Eds.), *The production of reality* (pp. 546–549). Sage.

Huffington, A. S. (2016). *The sleep revolution: Transforming your life, one night at a time*. Harmony Books.

Ingravallo, F., Gnucci, V., Pizza, F., Vignatelli, L., Govi, A., Dormi, A., Pelotti, S., Cicognani, A., Dauvilliers, Y., & Plazzi, G. (2012). The burden of narcolepsy with cataplexy: How disease history and clinical features influence socio-economic outcomes. *Sleep Medicine*, *13*(10), 1293–1300. https://doi.org/10.1016/j.sleep.2012.08.002

Insurance Institute for Highway Safety. (2017, April). *Safety belts*. IIHS. http://www.iihs.org/iihs/topics/laws/safetybeltuse?topicName=Safety%20belts#tableData

Jaeger, G., Röjvik, A., & Berglund, B. (2015). Participation in society for people with a rare diagnosis. *Disability and Health Journal*, *8*(1), 44–50. https://doi.org/10.1016/j.dhjo.2014.07.004

James, S. A. (1994). John Henryism and the health of African-Americans. *Culture, Medicine and Psychiatry*, *18*(2), 163–182. https://doi.org/10.1007/BF01379448

Japp, P. M., & Japp, D. K. (2005). Desperately seeking legitimacy: Narratives of a biomedically invisible disease. In L. M. Harter, P. M. Japp, & C. S. Beck (Eds.), *Narratives, health, and healing: Communication theory, research and practice* (pp. 107–130). Lawrance Erlbaum Associates.

Riviera Drew, J. A. (2015). Disability, poverty and material hardship since the passage of the ADA. *Disability Studies Quarterly, 35*(3), N. P.

Rothstein, R. (2017). *The color of law: A forgotten history of how our government segregated America*. Liveright Publishing Corporation.

Rubin, H. J., & Rubin, I. (2012). *Qualitative interviewing: The art of hearing data* (3rd ed.). Sage.

Sagaspe, P., Micoulaud-Franchi, J.-A., Coste, O., Léger, D., Espié, S., Davenne, D., Lopez, R., Dauvilliers, Y., & Philip, P. (2019). Maintenance of Wakefulness Test, real and simulated driving in patients with narcolepsy/hypersomnia. *Sleep Medicine*, *55*, 1–5. https://doi.org/10.1016/j.sleep.2018.02.009

Samuels, E. J. (2015). Passing. In R. Adams, B. Reiss, & D. Serlin (Eds.), *Keywords for disability studies* (pp. 135–136). New York University Press.

Schalk, S. D. (2022). *Black disability politics*. Duke University Press.

Scheiber, N. (2015, November 2). Fake Cover Letters Expose Discrimination Against Disabled. *The New York Times*. http://www.nytimes.com/2015/11/02/upshot/fake-cover-letters-expose-discrimination-against-disabled.html

Schutz, H., Walther, B. W., & Leonhard-Weigand, D. (2013). Intra-night sleep perception in patients with sleep disorders. In N. T. Oniani (Ed.), *Neurobiology of emotions, mind and sleep-wakefulness cycle* (pp. 47–55). Tbilisi.

Scott, J.-A. (2015). Narrative Performance Research: Co-Storying "Almost Passing." *Departures in Critical Qualitative Research, 4*(3), 70–91. JSTOR Journals. https://doi.org/10.1525/dcqr.2015.4.3.70

Sforza, E., Saint Martin, M., Thomas, T., Collet, P., Garet, M., Barthélémy, J. C., & Roche, F. (2017). Reply to "Letter to the Editor: Physical activity differently affects bone mineral density in obstructive sleep apnea at different age." *Sleep Medicine*, *32*, 274. https://doi.org/10.1016/j.sleep.2016.11.005

Shakespeare, T. (2006). The social model of disability. In L. J. Davis (Ed.), *The disability studies reader* (2nd ed., pp. 197–204). Routledge.

Siegel, J. M. (2000). Narcolepsy. *Scientific American*, *282*(1), 76–81. https://doi.org/10.1038/scientificamerican0100–76

Silberman, S. (2016). *Neurotribes: The legacy of autism and the future of neurodiversity.* Avery.

Simons, D., & Charis, C. (2010). *The invisible gorilla: And other ways our intuitions deceive us*. The Invisible Gorilla. http://www.theinvisiblegorilla.com/videos.html

Sleepy Sarah Elizabeth (Director). (2014, July 7). *What narcolepsy really looks like. Spoiler alert—It sucks.* https://www.youtube.com/watch?v=1PuvXpv0yDM

Smith, J. (2019). *From the back of the bus to the front of the classroom: My thirty-year journey as a Black and blind professor*. Monday Creek Publishing.

Smith, J. A., & Osborn, M. (2015). Interpretive Phenomenological Analysis. In J. A. Smith (Ed.), *Qualitative psychology: A practical guide to research methods* (2nd ed., pp. 53–80). Sage.

Stewart, K. (2007). *Ordinary affects*. Duke University Press.

Swoboda, D. A. (2006). The social construction of contested illness legitimacy: A grounded theory analysis. *Qualitative Research in Psychology*, *3*(3), 233–251. https://doi.org/10.1191/1478088706qrp061oa

Temple, J. (2015). *American pain: How a young felon and his ring of doctors unleashed America's deadliest drug epidemic*. Lyons Press.

Thorpy, M. J., & Krieger, A. C. (2014). Delayed diagnosis of narcolepsy: Characterization and impact. *Sleep Medicine*, *15*(5), 502–507. https://doi.org/10.1016/j.sleep.2014.01.015

Tillmann, L. M. (1996). A secret life in a culture of thinness: Reflections on body, food, and bulimia. In C. Ellis & A. P. Bochner (Eds.), *Composing ethnography: Alternative forms of qualitative writing* (pp. 76–108). AltaMira.

Trotter, B. (2014). *Narcoleptic driver causes concern for Ellsworth police* [Article]. *Bangor Daily News* (ME). http://bangordailynews.com/2014/08/22/news/hancock/narcoleptic-driver-causes-concern-for-ellsworth-police/

Utley, M. J. (1995). *Narcolepsy: A funny disorder that's no laughing matter*. M. J. Utley.

Valeras, A. (2010). "We don't have a box": Understanding hidden disability identity utilizing narrative research methodology. *Disability Studies Quarterly*, *30*(3/4). http://dsq-sds.org/article/view/1267

van der Sluiszen, N. N. J. J. M., Urbanus, B., Lammers, G. J., Overeem, S., Ramaekers, J. G., & Vermeeren, A. (2021). On-the-road driving performance of patients with central disorders of hypersomnolence. *Traffic Injury Prevention*, *22*(2), 120–126. https://doi.org/10.1080/15389588.2020.1862804

Vereijken, F. R., Giesbers, S. A. H., Jahoda, A., & Embregts, P. J. C. M. (2022). Homeward bound: Exploring the motives of mothers who brought their offspring with intellectual disabilities home from residential settings during the COVID-19 pandemic. *Journal of Applied Research in Intellectual Disabilities, 35*(1), 150–159.

The Voice of the Patient: Narcolepsy (Patient-Focused Drug Development Initiative). (2014). [Final]. Center for Drug Evaluation and Research (CDER) and U.S. Food and Drug Administration (FDA). https://www.fda.gov/downloads/ForIndustry/UserFees/PrescriptionDrugUserFee/UCM402907.pdf

Walker, N. (2013). Throw Away the Master's Tools: Liberating Ourselves from the Pathology Paradigm [Blog]. *Neurocosmopolitanism: Nick Walker's Notes on Neurodiversity, Autism, and Cognative Liberty*. http://neurocosmopolitanism.com/throw-away-the-masters-tools-liberating-ourselves-from-the-pathology-paradigm/

Wamsley, E., Donjacour, C. E. H. M., Scammell, T. E., Lammers, G. J., & Stickgold, R. (2014). Delusional confusion of dreaming and reality in narcolepsy. *Sleep*, *37*(2), 419–422. https://doi.org/10.5665/sleep.3428

Watkins, T. (2017). *A sick life: TLC 'n me: Stories from on and off the stage*. Rodale.

Watzlawick, P., Bavelas, J. B., & Jackson, D. D. (2014). *Pragmatics of human communication: A study of interactional patterns, pathologies, and paradoxes*. W. W. Norton & Company.

Wendell, S. (1996). *The rejected body: Feminist philosophical reflections on disability*. Routledge.

Wilenius, L., & Partinen, M. (2020). Attention-Deficit/Hyperactivity Disorder patients may have undiagnosed narcolepsy. *Cureus*, *12*(6). https://doi.org/10.7759/cureus.8436

Wilkerson, I. (2020). *Caste: The origins of our discontents* (1st ed.). Random House.

Wolf-Meyer, M. J. (2012). *The slumbering masses: Sleep, medicine, and modern American life*. University of Minnesota Press.

Wolf-Meyer, M. (2013). Editorial introduction: Alertness, or the other side of sleep. *Anthropology of Consciousness*, *24*(2), 93–95. https://doi.org/10.1111/anoc.12015

Wolf-Meyer, M. (2014). Therapy, remedy, cure: Disorder and the spatiotemporality of medicine and everyday life. *Medical Anthropology*, *33*(2), 144–159. https://doi.org/10.1080/01459740.2013.792812

Won, C., Mahmoudi, M., Qin, L., Purvis, T., Mathur, A., & Mohsenin, V. (2014). The impact of gender on timeliness of narcolepsy diagnosis. *Journal of Clinical Sleep Medicine*, *10*(1), 89–96. https://doi.org/10.5664/jcsm.3370

Woods-Giscombé, C. L. (2010). Superwoman schema: African American women's views on stress, strength, and health. *Qualitative Health Research*, *20*(5), 668–683. https://doi.org/10.1177/1049732310361892

Woods-Giscombé, C. L., Allen, A. M., Black, A. R., Steed, T. C., Li, Y., & Lackey, C. (2019). The Giscombe Superwoman Schema Questionnaire: Psychometric properties and associations with mental health and health behaviors in african american women. *Issues in Mental Health Nursing*, *40*(8), 672–681. https://doi.org/10.1080/01612840.2019.1584654

World Health Organization & World Bank (Eds.). (2011). *World report on disability*. World Health Organization.

Young, B. (2013). *Transcript of FDA Narcolepsy Public Meeting on Patient-Focused Drug Development*. Food and Drug Administration (FDA) & Center for Drug Evaluation and Research (CDER). https://www.fda.gov/downloads/ForIndustry/UserFees/PrescriptionDrugUserFee/UCM377107.pdf

Zamarian, L., Högl, B., Delazer, M., Hingerl, K., Gabelia, D., Mitterling, T., Brandauer, E., & Frauscher, B. (2014). Subjective deficits of attention, cognition and depression in patients with narcolepsy. *Sleep Medicine*, *16*(1), 45–51. https://doi.org/10.1016/j.sleep.2014.07.025

Index

About the Author

Nicole Eugene is Assistant Professor of Communication at the University of Houston-Victoria. She received her PhD from Ohio University in communication studies, her MA is from Bowling Green State University in American cultural studies and she studied sociology and art at Spelman College. She is an interdisciplinary scholar, a disability advocate, and a scholar-artist. She is the winner of numerous awards and her work has been supported by Ohio Humanities, a state affiliate of the National Endowment for the Humanities. Her research focuses on exploring hidden disabilities—often neurological disabilities—using either interpretive qualitative methods, autoethnography, or cultural studies. Nicole Eugene has published several articles and chapters, including peer-reviewed articles in *Howard Journal of Communications*, *Kaleidoscope: A Graduate Journal of Qualitative Communication Research*, and *Callaloo: A Journal of African Diaspora Arts and Letters*.

www.ingramcontent.com/pod-product-compliance
Ingram Content Group UK Ltd.
Pitfield, Milton Keynes, MK11 3LW, UK
UKHW041838031026
15587UKWH00002B/853

9 781666 913187